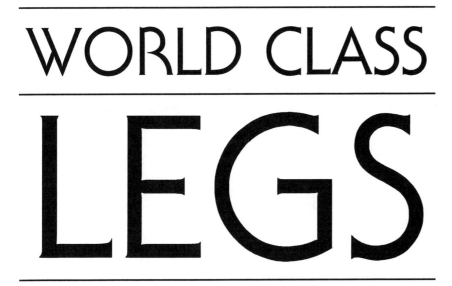

WORLD CLASS
LEGS

THE EFFECTIVE SIX-WEEK PROGRAM
TO SHAPING YOUR
LEGS, BUTT, AND THIGHS

by FELIX SCHMITT
and CYNTHIA TIVERS

A Fireside Book
Published by Simon & Schuster
New York   London   Toronto   Sydney   Tokyo   Singapore

F

FIRESIDE
Rockefeller Center
1230 Avenue of the Americas
New York, New York 10020

Designed by Irving Perkins Assoc.
Manufactured in the United States of America

1   3   5   7   9   10   8   6   4   2

Library of Congress Cataloging-in-Publication Data
Schmitt, Felix.
World class legs : the effective six-week program to shaping your
legs, butt and thighs / by Felix Schmitt and Cynthia Tivers.
p.   cm.
"A Fireside book."
1. Exercise for women.   2. Leg.   3. Beauty, Personal.   I. Tivers,
Cynthia.   II. Title.
GV482.S35   1994
613.7'045—dc20   93-5946
CIP
ISBN: 0-671-87025-4

Photographs by Richard Bomersheim

To my loving parents, Bella and William Kandelman, who have taught me better than the rest, loved me unconditionally, and honored me with their pride.

—Cynthia Tivers

I believe the best things in my life have come to me through my Lord and Savior Jesus Christ. For all that I thank Him. Then to Nancy, my best friend, teacher and supporter and to Perry, Hana, and Charles, God's most precious blessing to me and to Peter Schmittdiel, who taught me so well how to serve.

—Felix Schmitt

"His legs are pillars of alabaster, set on bases of fine gold."

—Song of Solomon, 5:15

ACKNOWLEDGMENTS

The authors would like to thank all the people who have contributed their time, talent, and toil to the making of this book. Without their support we wouldn't have a leg to stand on.

Thanks to Stan Corwin, whose insight, foresight, and intelligence started us rolling; Kara Leverte, our encouraging editor, whose perception has proved invaluable; and Richard Bomersheim, our talented photographer, whose eye and taste and good nature have made our images not only beautiful but inspiring.

And thanks to our beautiful World Class models: Nancy Norby (who delivered her third baby three months before these photos were taken), Julie Burgess Jacobsen, Deborah Kinsella, Dale Harimoto, and Martha Clark; and to Isabelle Voyat and Dance France for their World Class fashions.

The authors would like to add a special thanks to Lydia Bach for opening the wonderful door to Lotte's world.

CONTENTS

INTRODUCTION

At Sunset Plaza Fitness, we've trained thousands of women of all shapes and sizes to follow a simple exercise routine that has changed the look of their legs dramatically.

Since the Sunset Plaza Fitness Studio is located in the heart of one of Los Angeles' chicest neighborhoods, many of our clients have been celebrities, international models, world class athletes, and, frankly, some of the most well-heeled ladies in town. But the majority of our clients don't start out with superstar legs and model butts. They come here to get them. They're career women and mommies. The one thing all our students have in common—no matter what their background or their age—is the desire to look and feel their best. They want what we can promise: World Class Legs.

The Sunset Plaza Fitness Workout is ballet based. Starting with an emphasis on posture and form and the use of balletic positions, we've modified the key components of ballet to achieve the long and lean look ballet dancers are known for *without* the arduous training ballet dancers must endure.

Our method is an outgrowth of our training in the Lotte Berk method. Miss Berk, a ballerina, suffered injury to her spine and was forced to curtail her career. So, about thirty years ago, she developed exercises that used ballet postures that could be done in a limited way by people not trained as dancers. We started with her method and then, by extrapolating from her exercises, we invented our own workout. It's the workout you'll be using to shape your own World Class Legs.

If you devote half an hour, at least three times a week, to our workout, you'll lose inches off your thighs and you'll boost your butt higher than it's been since you were a kid. That's a promise. And the more you do our workout, the faster and better the results.

Our workout asks you to focus on postural awareness which goes beyond the time you spend doing our exercises and extends into the rest of your life. You're not going to just change your muscles with us, you're going to develop a dancer's attitude that will change the way you stand, the way you move, the way you hold yourself at all times.

When we ask you to lift your chest, move your shoulders back, keep your chin up, your pelvis tucked and your tummy in, we're asking you to concentrate on the key components that will keep you posturally correct throughout the day. That correct posture will help you carry your body proudly and that's an attitude we think you deserve.

Of course, we want to remind you . . . since you have the desire for World Class Legs, just make sure you're in world class health. Before you start our program, consult your physician. Tell your doctor you plan on working out with us and ask your physician's advice.

CHAPTER ONE

WORLD CLASS LEGS

If you were asked to name the group of women who have the best-shaped legs, chances are you'd think of ballet dancers. Ballet dancers spend years perfecting their form. Our exercises are as close as nondancers will ever get to working in ballet. But we've put another slant on ballet's primary movements that allows greater results. And with our method you don't have to spend years at the ballet barre; you can spend just weeks to get legs that are shaped and stretched to ballet perfection.

TAKING CONTROL

Most women say they feel least in touch with their lower bodies. And with good reason. For women, lower-body fat is the hardest to lose. It's stubborn and lazy fat. Lower-body fat doesn't move in and out of fat cells as readily as fat in other parts of the body. And thighs and butts have traditionally been the toughest to shape. But, over the years, we've developed a successful way to put you in touch with those trouble spots and, most importantly, to give you *control* over them.

Visualization is the key here. Close your eyes for a moment. Visualize your body. What do you see? Starting from the waist down . . . chances are you'll see a butt that's fallen far from its starting position. We all started out with behinds that were high and round. How about your thighs? Have you accumulated inches of fat? Have your muscles started to sag and become shapeless? And what about your knees? Have they become so padded that they drag down the look of your legs?

Now, open your eyes and look at the picture of the woman in Figure 1.1. Do you think you can get your legs to look anything close to what hers look like? We think you can. It's true, nature has handed you a blueprint, but now you're in for a remodeling. And we're going to show you how to take control of the reduction site. Develop a mental picture of what you want your own legs to look like. Take some time to work on that image. To get some ideas, thumb through this book and check out the shape of the legs you see. Think about your own legs. Wouldn't you like to drop the fat, shape the muscles, and develop a long, lean look? You can do it instantly in your mind. Go ahead, picture your legs in their ultimately beautiful shape. You want to etch that picture in your mind's eye. Memorize it. Carry it with you. Everywhere. Use it as motivation to exercise—especially on those days when you "just don't feel like it."

Use your desire for World Class Legs to override your desire for fattening foods. Every time you get the urge for chocolate cake or fried chicken, for instance, instead of picturing the food in your mind, pull out that mental picture of your great legs. If you eat fatty foods you'll sabotage your success in reaching your goal. Before you put anything into your mouth *stop* and *think*. What will that piece of food do to my mental picture? The promise of your image of World Class Legs becoming reality should help you control your eating habits and maintain your exercise program. Remember, you can become just as attached to exercise and feeling good as you are to tasting rich foods.

Once you start to see actual results from your work, and we promise you will, you'll feel your control working. You'll feel motivated to *stay* in control and get those World Class Legs.

Within six weeks your thighs will be thinner by two to three

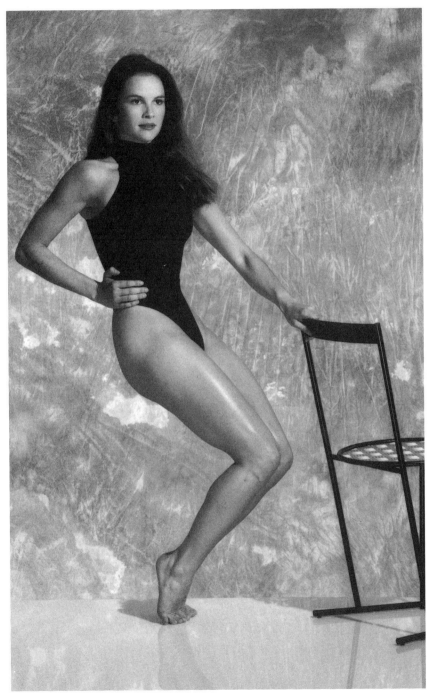

Figure 1.1 World Class Legs

inches in diameter. And they'll be shapelier, too. Your butt will be lifted and shaped in a round, firm way; your stomach will flatten and your waistline will lose at least two inches. Your entire lower body will look thinner and more elongated.

By now, if you're feeling overwhelmed by the prospect of working toward World Class Legs, put this book down for a while and think about what you really want. You see, you must believe you can take control. We know the results are possible. We've seen dramatic results hundreds of times in our clients. We believe you can get the same results. We want you to stick with us in this. We're about to share our leg-shaping secrets with you.

We'll give you an overall plan for fitness with simple ideas you can integrate easily into your daily life. And we'll make sure the exercise routines that you'll follow will make sense to you and your life-style. By understanding how you're working, you'll have better control over why and when you're working. Remember, taking control is the key here.

You'll find that not only will you lose inches in six weeks but since we're the *ultimate* tone and shape program you'll have the prettiest legs possible.

THE SEAT OF POWER

Your butt is the seat of your body's power. However, it takes a long time for most women to get in touch with their gluteus maximus because for most women their butts are so out of condition they can't even find the muscles to contract—a motion that's critical for our method. When you learn our techniques for controlling your rear end, you'll be able to take that floppy butt and make it fly. Not only will the shape of your bottom improve but your posture will, too.

Try this exercise and see what we mean. Stand up and put your hands on your butt. Hold it while you squeeze both cheeks together. Feel it pinching? Now tilt your pelvis up a little. (*This movement is a key one for our exercises, as you'll see a little later.*) Squeeze harder. Feel your butt tightening? Don't stop. Squeeze harder. It won't hurt. It will actually feel good. Even if your muscles are buried under layers of fat, you'll still feel the strength that's underneath. That strength from your butt is going to help you develop World Class Legs. We guarantee it.

By strengthening your seat you'll get more control over your upper thighs and hips. And you'll strengthen your lower lumbar region (your lower back: the area covering your bottom ten vertebrae) which will give your entire body more flexibility. That means you'll not only feel better but you'll look more youthful, too. And people will notice. Many of our clients have told us stories that prove World Class Legs can give you a World Class Attitude. Emotionally, that's quite a boost for anyone.

TAKING THE PRESSURE OFF

The key to our method of shaping and toning is the pelvic rotation or tuck. As you go through our exercise routine, the function of the tuck will become continually clearer to you. The tuck sets your body up to stretch at the same time your muscles strengthen.

A muscle worked without pelvic rotation looks different from one

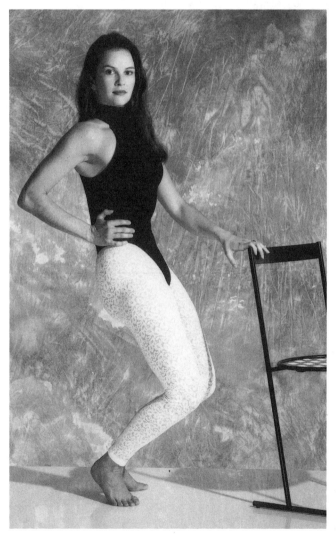

*Figure 1.2
The seat of
power*

which is rotated and stretched. It's like a partially tightened guitar string. It can only hit a flat note. But when the muscle becomes more extended in its stretch, it has more tone because there's more tension on the entire string. The tuck is the ticket to success for that longer, leaner look.

Try it once and you'll get some idea of what we mean. Use Figure 1.2 as your example. Stand with your hand on the back of a chair. Place your heels together and raise them about an inch off the floor. Without lowering your heels, bend your knees and lower at least an inch. Pay close attention to how your muscles feel. You should feel some pull on your quadriceps, the front of your thighs. Now stand up straight again. Keep your heels lifted but this time find your tuck. Rotate your pelvis forward and squeeze your buttocks together. Now lower again. Feel the difference? You will feel more stretching of the quadriceps *and* at the same time you're giving yourself more strength by controlling your butt, which is also being worked.

The pelvic rotation sets up your thighs, butt, stomach, and lower back for strength and flexibility, too. Our method is unique in that it's the only way to accomplish stretching and strengthening simultaneously. As you felt just now, doing the previous exercise, the pelvic rotation sets up a specific stretch in the quadriceps muscles and hamstrings.

At the same time the tuck is working your muscles, it's taking pressure off your lower back, which is typically a problem area for women. Most women carry tension in their lower backs, and that part of their bodies is generally inflexible. By using the tuck, you'll be increasing flexibility in your lower back. So when you utilize the tuck in exercises for your abdominal muscles, you'll be able to work more deeply and effectively.

FOOD FOR THOUGHT

We're about ready to start shaping up your body. But before we do, a word about your diet. *Fat.* That's the word. It's your enemy. If you modify your intake of fat grams to 30 percent of your caloric intake, you'll be on the road to better fitness. If you reduce your fat intake to 20 or 25 grams a day you'll reduce your weight. It's not the calories. It's the fat. And these days we're lucky. Many of the foods we buy in the supermarket have their fat content listed on their labels. Read them. If you have any doubts, don't buy it. You'll get used to living without excess fat in your body or on your body.

If you're looking for a specific diet designed to meet your particular tastes and life-style, a qualified nutritionist can help you plan a balanced low-fat diet.

And one more hint: *Drink water.* Lots of water. It provides oxygen and nutrients to your muscles. It cuts down on your feelings of hunger. It keeps flushing out your system. Remember: Waste not . . . waist not.

CHAPTER TWO

BASIC ANATOMY

Muscles. Everybody's got them. Yours may be hidden under a few layers of fat, but we're going to help you dig them out. Muscle can be shaped; fat keeps you shapeless. We want you to lose the fat, build muscle, then shape and tone it.

For every pound of fat you replace with muscle, you burn more calories. Muscle tissue burns more calories than fat cells do. The idea is to make your body more efficient at burning calories by building up your muscle-to-fat ratio. You can do this by sticking to a low-fat diet, doing an aerobic workout, and by strengthening your body's muscles with our workout.

Our six-week workout focuses on your lower body—where women have 80 percent of their body strength—but we are going to use your upper body in our routine, too. You'll be using your arms during the warm-up—first as a cardiovascular stimulus and second in push-ups to build upper-body strength and tone. After all, what good are World Class Legs if you can't use shapely arms to point to them with pride?

Let's take a little time here to get acquainted with the parts of the body we'll be concentrating on.

LOWER-BODY MUSCLES AND JOINTS

QUADRICEPS. The front of the thigh—which we will be working extensively—is called the quadriceps. The quadriceps is actually a group of four muscles that run down the front of the thigh to insert at the kneecap. They all work to extend the leg and to flex the thigh. The muscles work collectively to help keep the kneecap in place. The appearance of a woman's leg is mostly determined by the shape of her quadriceps. You're going to learn how to build the quad up and elongate it. Our exercises will also work the hips into shape.

ADDUCTORS. These are the inner-thigh muscles and, as far as exercise goes, they're the hardest for women to find. The adductors, which start at the pubic bone and go down to the side of the knee, work to flex the thigh, pull the leg in, and to keep the knees pulled together. Most standard exercises don't stretch the adductors but when you get into our workout, particularly in Second Position and in our "wall with the ball" work, you'll not only find those adductors and stretch them but you'll shape and tone them, too.

HAMSTRINGS. Three muscles in the back of the thigh which flex the knee, rotate the leg, and extend the hips. The hamstrings need elongation and strengthening in order to give the leg a long, lean look. Flexible hamstrings also contribute to a better-shaped butt.

GLUTEUS MAXIMUS. One of the largest muscles in the body and in most women it rests behind the hip joint. When we get through with you, your glut will never rest; it will always be squeezing and contracting, lifting the butt from where it intersects with the back of the thigh.

KNEES. Our workout will build strong and flexible ligaments and tendon support. We work the muscles that attach to the knees on all sides. We strengthen the muscles that hold the kneecap in place. Throughout our exercises you'll feel a stretch in the front of your knee. You'll be strengthening a weak area. Everyone wants shapely knees extending into the thigh. And you're going to get them.

FEET. As you get older, your feet spread. And most women don't have real strength in their arches. Our exercises will build up the muscles around your metatarsals. The metatarsals are the long bones that make up part of the arch and the ball of your foot. With our exercises, the muscles in your feet will contract rather than expand. We've even had clients tell us they've gone down half a shoe size because they've improved the muscle condition of their feet.

UPPER-BODY MUSCLES AND BONES

The upper-body muscles that we'll primarily work on strengthening are:

DELTOIDS. These muscles are used mainly to raise the arm, as well as to flex, extend, and rotate the arm. We'll use them when we do our push-ups during the warm-up segment of the workout.

BICEPS. The muscles on the front of the upper arm. They act to flex the arm. They'll come into play in our push-ups.

TRICEPS. The muscles of the back of the upper arm. They act to extend the arm and forearm. These muscles tend to get flabby on women as they age. We'll work on shaping them up with our tricep push-ups that come in the third week.

PECTORALIS. This fan-shaped muscle runs along the breastbone to the cartilage connecting the upper ribs to the breastbone. The pectoralis gets involved with all movement of the upper arm. You'll feel it build as we work on our push-ups.

RECTUS ABDOMINUS. The long, powerful muscle that runs from the fifth, sixth, and seventh ribs down to the pubic bone. This

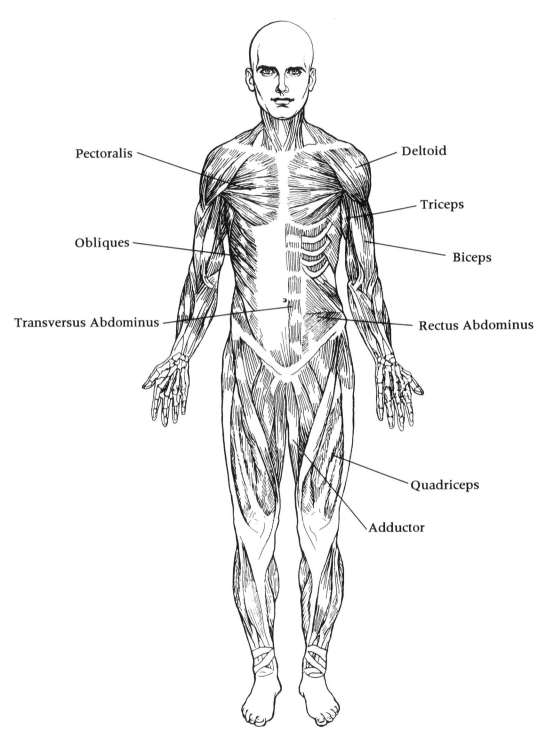

Pectoralis

Deltoid

Triceps

Obliques

Biceps

Transversus Abdominus

Rectus Abdominus

Quadriceps

Adductor

From the front—muscles: what we're working

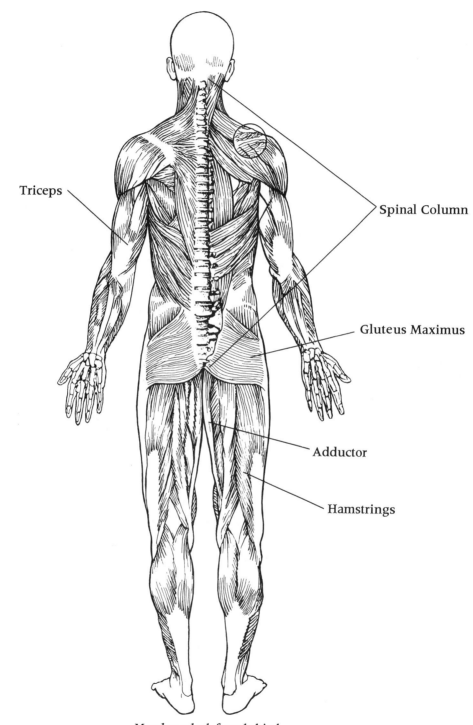

Triceps

Spinal Column

Gluteus Maximus

Adductor

Hamstrings

Muscles: a look from behind

muscle pulls your torso toward your lower body during sit-ups. You'll also use it in your pelvic tucks.

OBLIQUES. These muscles fuse with the fibrous tissue covering the rectus abdominus and form a girdle around the abdomen. The internal and external obliques rotate the trunk of your body and help you flex your torso. You'll feel them working in the warm-up.

TRANSVERSUS ABDOMINUS. This is the muscle that runs across the midsection of your abdomen and helps you pull in your tummy throughout our entire set of exercises.

THE SPINAL COLUMN. You have twenty-four vertebrae which are stacked and separated by cartilage and soft cushions in your spinal column. There are interacting muscles which run on both sides of the spinal column. They're responsible for rotating the lower back. They also extend and bend the lower back sideways. Whereas most exercises, particularly aerobic exercise, compress the spinal column, our workout decompresses the spine by stretching it.

The pelvic rotations that are the key to the effectiveness of all our exercises work to strengthen the spine. As you tuck, you push up the lower lumbar area, which helps give you greater flexibility and muscle strength.

By tucking up the pelvic area, we take pressure off the pelvic girdle, giving greater strength in the back and flexibility in the lower back. Our exercises give muscle balance in the lower back region. You'll find you're less prone to lower-back injury after you've stretched and strengthened with us.

REDEFINING YOUR MUSCLES

Now that you've got an idea of the names, placement, and function of the muscles we'll be working on, add two words to the description of those muscles: long and lean.

We will work the muscles in specific motions that will contract your leg and butt muscles as you're stretching them. The end result will be to redefine your muscles to look long and lean.

Now we're going to ask you to do something pretty brave. Strip down to your underwear and stand in front of a mirror. First look at your thighs. Can you find your quadriceps? Are they defined or are they hidden? Put your hand over your knee where it meets the start of your thigh. Now pull up on that muscle. You may not be able to see it tighten yet but you will feel it. That's your starting point. Run your hand up your thigh, pulling the skin up as you go. That's where you're going to end up. From here on, that muscle's going to lift as it gets tighter and stronger. You're going to build it up off the bone and it's going to take a new shape that's longer and leaner.

Now, turn so you can see your gluteus maximus. Does it hang so it touches the top of your hamstrings? Squeeze it as you pull up on both sides. See the separation between the butt and thigh? That's going to be your look within six weeks.

So, are you ready to redefine your muscles? OK, let's get started.

CHAPTER THREE

THE WARM-UP

We have six weeks of workouts designed to progressively strengthen and shape your muscles. Each week's workout will be explained in detail in a chapter devoted to that week's work. You may want to read through an entire chapter first so you will know what to expect that week. Then return to the exercises and use the book for reference.

WARMING UP

Our goal in the next six weeks is to burn fat off your body while we're building shapely legs, butts, and thighs. Cardiovascular training is where we start.

Aerobic exercises improve the operating strength of your heart, lungs, and vascular system. Exercises are considered aerobic if they are performed over prolonged periods of time and have repeated and continuous movements. Some examples are walking, running, swimming, cross-country skiing, step routines, stair climbing. They all increase your heart and lung capacity. The better your lungs inhale oxygen, the more strongly your heart pumps blood and the more efficiently oxygen is delivered throughout the body, making more oxygen available to your muscles to use for energy. That's good news because fat needs oxygen to burn and aerobic exercise uses fat as its major fuel.

With aerobic exercise your stored fat will burn off in bigger amounts. And not only that, aerobic exercise preserves muscle, ensuring that the calories you're burning will be fat calories.

A word of caution: Don't embark on a rigorous exercise regimen without consulting your physician. Your best bet is always to start slowly and progress. It's the plan we have for developing World Class Legs. You'll see the exercise program gain in intensity as you go through the six weeks detailed in this book.

While our workout itself is not aerobic—it's muscle shaping and toning—we think the benefits of a good cardiovascular workout are as important to your overall well-being as to your ability to perform our exercise routine. We recommend a minimum of thirty minutes of aerobic exercise three times a week, alternating days with our workout, which should take thirty to forty minutes per session. For maximum results, you can follow your thirty minutes of aerobics by our workout five times a week. But if you can't do the cardiovascular training before you do our workout, you must at least do our warm-up for five to ten minutes.

Remember, never work your muscles without warming up first. Cold muscles are prone to injury.

TARGETING YOUR HEART RATE

It is possible to exercise so hard you get a negative effect. Too much exertion leaves you gasping for the oxygen your muscles are demanding. If you're overworking, your body can't deliver that oxygen, which in turn exhausts your muscles. Overexertion tears down lean muscle mass which is vital to your body.

Your heart, for instance, is a muscle, so it's important that you know what your heart rate should be to be effective during exercise. That is your target heart range or the minimum rate at which your heart should be beating to get the optimum aerobic conditioning effect.

Your target heart range is 75 percent of your maximum heart rate. Here's how you figure out what those numbers are.

The formula for maximum heart rate is 220 minus your age. So if you're forty years old, your maximum heart rate (or your pulse count per minute) is 180. Now multiply this number by 75 percent. It's 135 beats per minute, which is what your pulse rate should be after you exercise.

Here's how you take your heart rate. With your index and middle fingers, find your pulse on the side of your neck at your collar bone. Count the number of beats for ten seconds and multiply by six. That's the number of beats your heart takes in one minute.

You should check your heart rate five minutes into your exercise and then again at five-minute intervals. If at any time you find your heart rate is more than your target heart range—*slow down.* Don't stop. Keep your feet moving when you check your rate.

Look at the chart that follows and see how many beats your heart should be taking to work within your target heart range.

TARGET HEART RANGE CHART

Age	Beats per 10 Seconds During Exercise
20–25	20–28
25–30	20–27
30–35	19–26
35–40	19–25
40–45	18–25
45–50	18–24
50–55	17–23
55–60	16–21

Your thirty minutes of aerobics should break down to a five-minute warm-up, which is what you need to get you to your target heart range. Then you'll work at your target heart range for twenty-two minutes, followed by a three-minute cool-down. If you want to get into a fat-burning phase, you can add another fifteen to thirty minutes of exercise, but you should do it at a much lower intensity—40 percent of your maximum heart rate or, if we use the forty-year-old's numbers, you work at a target heart rate of seventy-two.

You'll burn more fat riding an exercise bike for sixty minutes at 40 percent of your target heart range than you will by training at 75 percent of your maximum heart rate for twenty-two minutes. Besides, it's easier to pedal for one hour at forty rpm than for thirty minutes at ninety rpm. Remember, it's duration, rather than intensity, that will help you burn fat.

But we don't care how much you step, or run, or do aerobic exercises, you won't have World Class Legs that look long and lean, attached to a butt that looks round and high, unless you work at shaping and toning with the exercises you'll be mastering in the next six weeks.

So, if you're ready to heat it up, let's start at the beginning—with the fuel to feed your workout.

INTERNAL COMBUSTION

Eat at least one hour before you exercise. It gives your body a chance to metabolize your food so it can be used as an efficient energy source.

Your pre-exercise meal should consist primarily of complex carbohydrates (a slice of whole wheat toast, half a grapefruit) for their longer-lasting energy, and some protein (half a cup of nonfat yogurt or an egg white) which is good muscle food. Stay away from sugars and fat because neither burns efficiently and, in fact, they can reduce your energy level.

If you work out at the end of the day, don't do it on an empty stomach. Eat a low-sugar, low-fat bran muffin or a slice of whole wheat bread about an hour before your session. These complex carbohydrates will give you accessible energy.

Exercising on an empty stomach isn't wise. Your body needs the energy provided by the carbohydrates and protein to work efficiently. And *never* exercise without afterwards replenishing the water your body loses.

THE TOOLS

The women who work out at Sunset Plaza Fitness tell us they like working out in leotards and tights. They're comfortable and they allow you to monitor your muscles' movements better than if you wear sweats or loose-fitting clothes. You can start out with a T-shirt or a sweatshirt over your tights until you get warm, then discard it so your view is unobstructed.

It's best to work out in front of a mirror. That way you can check yourself for form. Once we get into the workout we'll be using a ballet barre. That's what we have in our studio. But you don't need a barre at home to do our exercises. You can use the back of a chair or sofa or even a doorknob. In fact, you can exercise in your bathroom, where there is sure to be a mirror and a countertop, towel rack, or doorknob you can hold on to. You'll also need a rug, carpeting, or some kind of padding for those times when you work on the floor.

Wherever you work out, you'll want it to be near your cassette deck or CD player. We think music is a key component of our entire workout. It makes the workout fun because music helps give you energy, it excites you, and motivates you to move.

You need music with a steady beat; we suggest a moderate rhythm of about 120 beats per minute. Try artists like the Pointer Sisters, Michael Jackson, Hammer, Whitney Houston, or Seal. These are only suggestions, though. Go with your favorites, since you and these artists will be companions throughout your workout.

You can combine artists by making your own tapes for variety. That way, you won't have to stop to change the music. The music will provide you with momentum and you'll find the time will go faster and more enjoyably.

HAVE A BALL

The only piece of equipment that you will need for our routine is a ball. You can use anything from a kickball to a utility yard ball. It should be about twelve inches in diameter—no larger than a basketball and no smaller than a volleyball. It should feel substantial (a beach ball is too thin) because it will have to endure pressure from the squeezing motion of your thighs and offer some resistance to your thigh muscles in order to be effective.

ONWARD AND UPWARD

We'll start with our ten-minute warm-up. This part of the workout will stay consistent throughout the six weeks, although we will add push-ups in the second week and gradually increase the number of them you do as time goes by.

None of our exercises, from the warm-up through the cool-down stretch, are jarring or ballistic. Our workout is orthopedically correct. There's no rushing through the moves, no bouncing, no trying to keep up with a tempo that overwhelms your ability to stay in touch with your muscles. We leave you less room for mistakes. The steady pace at which we work will maximize your mind-body interaction.

No matter what exercise you're doing, your form is important. Your posture is critical. We'll keep reminding you. And if at any time you feel you need to readjust, check yourself against the photographs and reset.

Put on your music. Stand in front of a mirror, with your hands extended in front of you. Stand with your back straight and shoulders down. Keep your arms extended from your shoulders. We're going to start with leg lifts.

Let's try the movement first. Lift your right leg, with your knee slightly bent. Lift it as close to your right hand as possible and lower it. Count one. Now do the other leg. Count two. (Figure 3.1)

You're going to do sixty of these leg lifts, alternating legs. To the music . . .

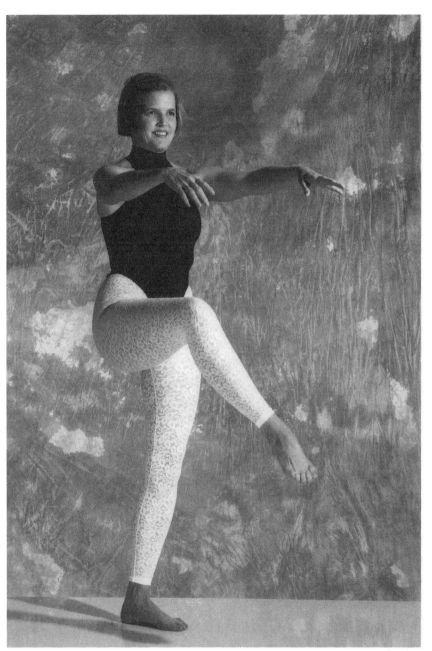

Figure 3.1

To continue: Keep lifting your legs. Now move your arms out to your sides at shoulder level, and lift them up over your head and back down to shoulder height. You raise your arms during one leg lift and then lower them during the next. Keep counting your leg lifts and do sixty more—right, left, right, left—combined with this up-and-down arm movement. (Figure 3.2)

Figure 3.2

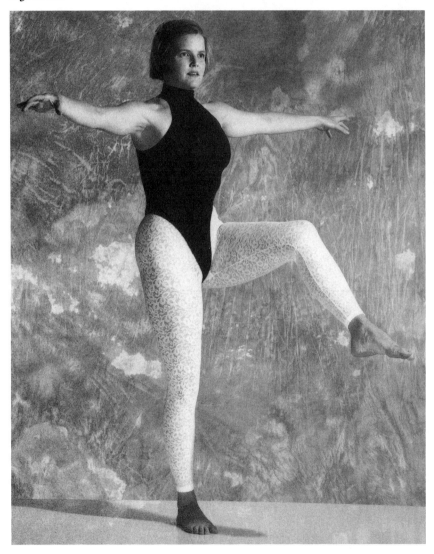

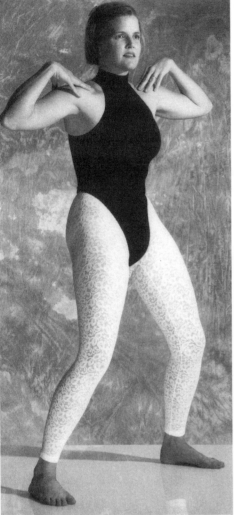

Figure 3.3 Central posture

Now stand in place and put your hands on your shoulders with your elbows wide and knees slightly bent. Make sure your feet are shoulder-width apart. Squeeze your butt and rotate your pelvis forward and up. Check it out. This is the tuck we'll be doing in the rest of the book. It's our central posture. (Figure 3.3)

Keep that tuck and bend to your right with your elbow pointing down toward the floor. Come back up to center and bend left. Each cycle of side, center, side is a count of one. Do it twenty times.

NOW, STRETCH

Bend over with your hands down as close to the floor as you can get them. Keep your weight forward on the balls of your feet. Your knees should be straight here only if it's comfortable. If you have back problems, start with your knees slightly bent and keep them bent throughout the rest of this stretching exercise. (Figure 3.4)

Remember, flexibility will increase with your count, so the stretch will get deeper the longer you hold it. Hold this first stretch for a count of thirty. *Do not bounce!* This should be a slow, gradual move and hold.

Now, without moving your hips, and keeping your weight forward on the balls of your feet, take your right hand and reach to your left knee. Your left arm should be extended up overhead behind you. Bring your nose toward your left knee and hold for a count of thirty. Not a quick thirty—a slow thirty. Don't lift up, just move over to your right with your nose pointed toward your right knee and your left hand holding your right knee. Your right arm extends overhead and behind you. Hold for a count of thirty. (Figure 3.5)

Slowly, bend your knees and sit down on the floor for a straddle stretch that will stretch out your back and your legs. Make sure your legs are flat on the floor, your toes pointed up to the ceiling, and your legs as wide apart as you can hold them. (Figure 3.6)

Bend your torso down to the floor between your legs and reach as far forward as you can. Hold for a count of thirty, being aware that your stretch will improve throughout the count and you can *slowly* crawl your fingers farther forward. Now move over along the floor to your left leg and place your torso over your leg. Your arms will rest on each side of that leg. Hold for a count of thirty and then repeat the motion over to your right leg and hold for a count of thirty.

You're now ready to start your World Class Legs Workout.

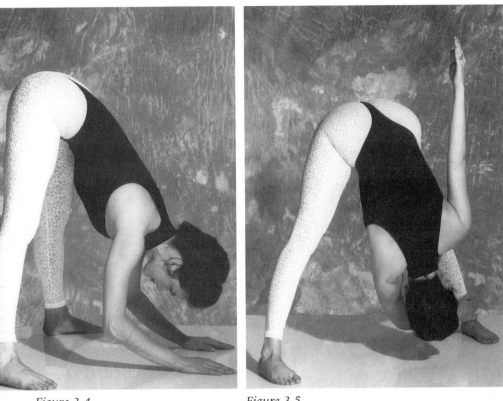

Figure 3.4   *Figure 3.5*

Figure 3.6 Straddle Stretch

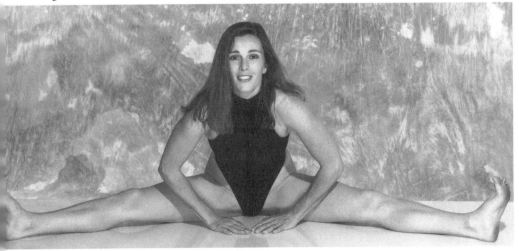

CHAPTER FOUR

WEEK ONE

THE BARRE

There's going to be a lot of talking going on inside your head for the next six weeks as you master the Workout for World Class Legs. Listen carefully to your "mind talk" and to your "body talk."

As you exercise, your body's going to tell you where you feel a muscle working hard—which can cause what we call "good" pain—or if you're doing something, like moving that muscle incorrectly, which will cause "bad" pain.

Your mind will send signals to your brain that will warn you to distinguish between the two. If, at any time, you feel discomfort, take a moment to determine if it's bad pain—if you feel like you're really hurting. If you're doing the exercises right, you'll feel a sensation unlike any you've ever had before. Your muscles will feel warm; they'll feel used, not abused; they'll feel stretched; and the muscles you're working will feel isolated from the other muscles in your body. These are all signs of "good" pain. Go with it. Don't run interference by using any pain as an excuse to stop. Distinguish between the bad pain and the good pain.

The only way you're going to build strength in your muscles is by pushing them to work. In the next few weeks your muscles will probably be working harder than they've ever worked before. And there will be times during your workout when your muscles will seem to scream "No!"

It happens with our clients. But the moment they say they can't do something, we remind them they can. When you hear that internal no, respond with yes. You *can* do it—we're sure of it.

OK, now that you're all fired up . . . let's move to the barre.

BALANCE AT THE BARRE

The first section of our workout is at the barre. You can use the back of a sofa, a dining room chair, the kitchen counter, or the towel rack in the bathroom. Whatever "barre" you use, its optimal height should be between waist and chest high. You don't want to lean on your barre. It's a balancing barre that will help you focus on your posture. You can't have balance without correct posture.

Put your "barre" in front of the mirror and stand sideways to the mirror so you can monitor your body's posture and movements while you hold the barre.

These exercises are very specific in their movements. Many of the moves are very subtle and, just like in ballet, balance is an integral part of our exercises. In addition, with good posture comes better breathing. So start by rotating your shoulders up, back, and down.

FIRST POSITION

Put your hand on your barre and place your heels together so they touch. Lift them one inch off the floor. The front of your feet should be no more than six inches apart.

Suck in your tummy, squeeze your gluteus maximus. Now scoop your pelvic girdle in an under-and-forward direction and hold it. Bend your knees about two inches. They should be bent directly out over your toes. This is your starting position. (Figure 4.1)

Release your tuck and tuck again by squeezing your seat hard. Be sure to focus on your upper body posture here. Your tendency will

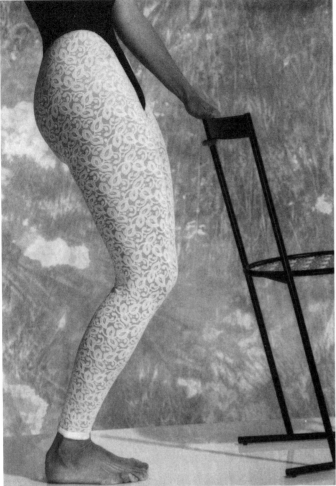

Figure 4.1
First Position

be to hunch your shoulders and slouch, so you watch yourself carefully in the mirror.

Now bend your knees another inch and tuck, release, and tuck and release. Loosen your squeeze when you release but don't stick your bottom out . . . stay in a tucked position. Bend your knees one more inch. This is your third level down. At this level, tuck and release three times. On your fourth tuck *hold* for a count of ten.

Lift back up to the first level. Remember, your knees are bent two inches at the first level. Now repeat two tucks at the first level, bend your knees an inch and do two tucks at the second level, and then go down to the third level for four tucks, and *hold* for a count of ten.

This hold will help you build strength. Make sure you keep your tuck. The tuck will make sure your entire gluteus muscle is involved so the exercise will be more effective.

Each repetition of this movement consists of two tucks at the first level, two tucks at the second level, and two tucks at the third level. Do five repetitions to complete one set.

Repeat the entire First Position set a second time.

STRETCHING IT OUT

You've been working your butt and your quadriceps by simultaneously contracting and stretching the muscles to build their strength. Now it's important to increase the stretch of your working muscles. The stretching will increase your flexibility and help shape your muscles into that longer, leaner look we're working toward.

The Standing Quadriceps Stretch is done at the barre. We'll start by stretching the left quad. Hold the barre with your right hand. Bend your right knee slightly—that's the standing leg—and then bend your left knee, reaching back to hold your left foot behind you with your left hand. (Figure 4.2)

Tuck your pelvis by squeezing your butt and rotating forward so the stretch of the quad is pulled back against your squeezing seat. The pelvic rotation locks the stretch in place and immediately engages the upper half of the quad so the muscle is stretched from the pubic bone down to the knee.

Don't pull your heel all the way to your seat. It overstretches the knee. Keep your heel out about three inches from your seat.

Make sure your shoulders are back and down. Hold for a count of twenty.

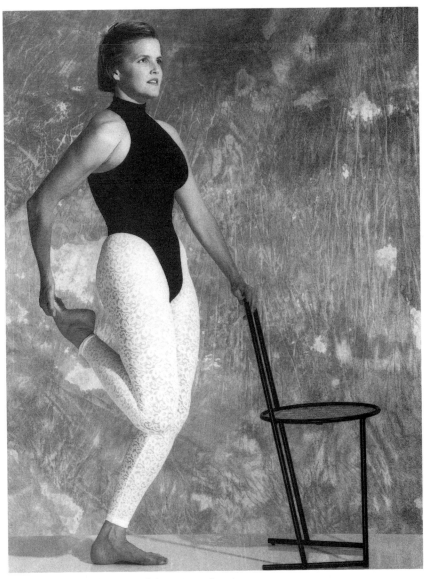

Figure 4.2 Standing Quadriceps Stretch

Switch legs. Hold the barre with your left hand. Bend your left knee slightly—the standing leg—then bend your right knee and take hold of your foot with your right hand and pull it back against your tuck.

Hold for a count of twenty.

SECOND POSITION

Once again, hold on to the barre. Place your feet shoulder-width apart, feet parallel, with your knees and your feet pointed straight ahead. This placement is called Second Position. Lift your heels at least one inch off the floor. (Figure 4.3) Suck in your tummy, tuck your pelvis, bend your knees two inches. That's your starting point in this position. Squeeze your butt hard and release. Tuck again at this level. Go down an inch to the second level and tuck and release twice. Lower another inch and tuck and release three times. On the fourth tuck *hold* for a count of ten.

Lift back up to the starting point, with your knees bent two inches and your pelvis tucked up and forward. Repeat this tucking and lowering exercise a total of five times to complete one set.

Do the Standing Quadriceps Stretch for both legs. (See Figure 4.2) Your quads will feel a little looser this time. That's good. Hold the stretch for a count of twenty on each leg. Check your posture. Make sure you're not hunched over. Breathe deeply.

Repeat the exercises five more times to complete a second set.

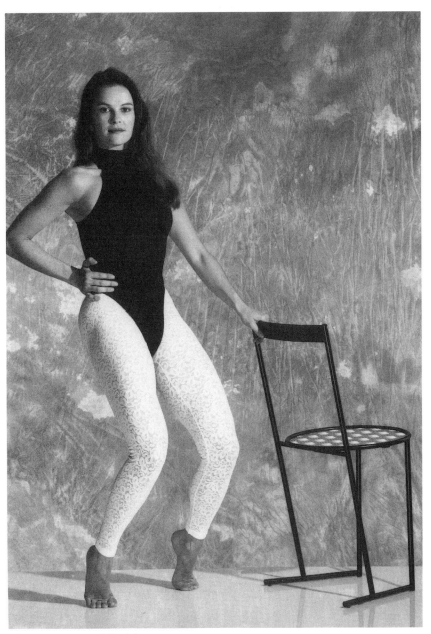

Figure 4.3 Second Position

HAVE A SEAT

Sit down on a firm chair. It can have a cushion but you want to be sure you don't sink into the chair. Sit at the edge of the seat and place the ball between your knees. Keep your feet apart, but hold the ball in place by applying pressure with your inner thighs. Sit up straight and keep your hands on either side of you. (Figure 4.4)

Squeeze that ball as hard as you can and hold it in the squeezed position for a count of three. The hold will activate your muscles quickly. Release the squeeze—but not the ball—then squeeze again and hold again for a count of three. Do this a total of thirty times for one set.

Repeat the set.

This exercise really wakes up your inner thigh muscles.

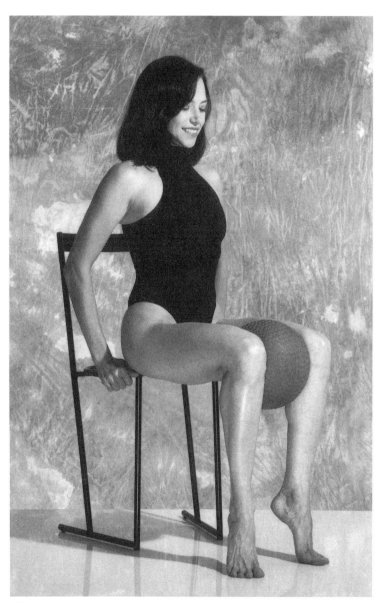

Figure 4.4

TO THE WALL

This next exercise will be done on the floor with your feet up against the wall. You'll want to do this while you lie on carpeting or a pad so you protect your back. Wear socks for this one so you don't stain or spot the wall.

Lie on your back on the floor with your knees bent and your feet parallel on the wall, shoulder-width apart. Start your pelvic rotation by squeezing your seat. Let the natural upward rotation of the pelvis take place. *Do not lift your lower back off the floor* by pushing with the front of your thighs or by lifting with your back. Keep your back on the floor and rotate the hips, pelvis, and buttocks by squeezing and lifting only your seat. (Figure 4.5)

Figure 4.5

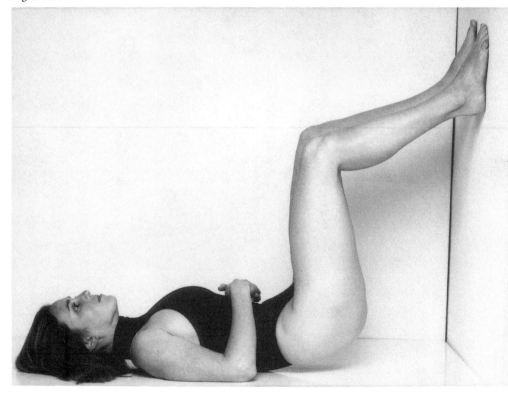

This is not a big movement. It's small and contained. The movement is: rotate your pelvis two times up and two times down. Keep this rhythm in your mind: Up, up. Down, down.

Do it slowly and methodically thirty times to complete one set. Then hug your knees to stretch out your gluteus maximus. Repeat the set. And again hug your knees.

This is a simple exercise, but don't underestimate its value. It seems very easy but if it's done correctly, it can be a really intense bun burner. And, at the same time, you're strengthening and flexing your lower back.

COOL-DOWN STRETCH

Now it's time for the ever-important cool-down. Every exercise session should start with a warm-up and end with a cool-down.

Stay on the floor and push away from the wall. Your muscles are warm now so they're ready to stretch. Lie on your back with both legs bent at the knee, feet flat on the floor. Lift your left leg and reach for your leg with both hands. (Figure 4.6)

If you're tight in your lower back area, reach just below the kneecap. If you have more flexibility, reach to your calf or ankle and pull your leg as close to your body as possible. Flex your foot and straighten your knee. You'll feel the stretch in your hamstring. Now

Figure 4.6

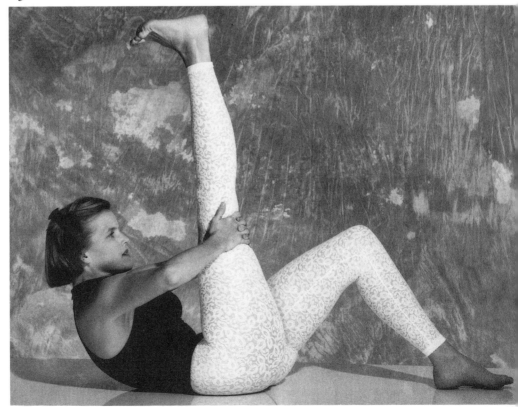

lift your head up toward the knee. Remember to keep your stomach pulled in. The stretch will go from the back of your knee, up your hamstring, to the insertion point or base of the butt. Pull to the point of feeling the stretch but if you feel pain, release your leg.

In a stretch, never go to a point where the pain is so uncomfortable it's unpleasant. Do go to the point of feeling activated.

Hold your left leg for a count of thirty. Then switch legs, repeat the stretch and hold for a count of thirty.

Congratulations! You've just completed your first Workout session.

Repeat this Workout at least three times during the week. Each time you go through it, you'll become more familiar with the positions. The work won't get easier but, as you become accustomed to it, you'll be more in touch with what's happening in your muscles with every contraction and stretch you take.

If, for any reason, you don't feel comfortable enough yet with these beginning exercises, feel free to repeat the exercises for another week before you move on to Week Two. You'll continue to get the benefits of the Workout as you learn the positions better.

CHAPTER FIVE

WEEK TWO

If you find you prefer exercising with a partner, make sure you choose someone who is not only dependable but who is at least as motivated as you are about owning a pair of World Class Legs. Exercising with someone else does have its advantages. Enthusiasm, for one thing, is contagious. A partner can be supportive and can encourage you to go that extra inch or do that one last push-up. Another person can also help you check your form and catch you if you drop your heels or round your chest when you should be standing up straight.

If you do decide to work out with another person, set a schedule to which you both can stick. If one of you can't make it, it's too easy to find an excuse not to exercise at all. No matter if you work alone or with someone else, once you get started, don't disrupt your rhythm. Don't miss a session—move it around in your schedule if you have to but never drop your workout time.

When you work out, work out. Don't stop between sets to take phone calls or to gossip with one another. Focus strictly on what you're doing. Remember, it's OK to stop and take a drink of water. But keep the water nearby and don't linger. You don't want to lose your momentum.

One of the advantages to our Workout is there are no fast moves, no quick starts or stops. You can move pretty much at your own pace. You don't have to worry that if you miss a beat you've missed a movement. So don't let anybody rush you through your Workout. Take your time and make sure you get it right.

Remember, when you get it right you get the reward and the World Class title.

REHEAT

Your second week will start with the same warm-up as Week One.

In short, do sixty Leg Lifts—right, left, for a total of thirty with your right and thirty with your left leg —with your hands stretched forward at shoulder level. (See Figure 3.1, page 35)

Move your arms to the side and up and down as you do sixty more Leg Lifts, alternating left and right.

With your hands on your shoulders and a pelvic tuck, bend your knees slightly. Bend your upper body to your right side with your right elbow pointing down. Come back up to center and then bend left, with your left elbow pointing down toward the floor. Repeat this movement of side, center, and side twenty times. (Figure 5.1)

NEW THIS WEEK: PUSH-UPS

Push-ups will help you get your heart rate going while you're building up your biceps and your pectoralis muscles—those are the chest muscles that can give your breasts a lift.

On your hands and knees, with your knees together and your hands shoulder-width apart, squeeze your butt, *tuck* your pelvis and pull in your abdominals to protect your back. Move your weight forward onto your arms. Fingertips should point straight ahead, shoulder-width apart. Bend the elbows slightly. (Figure 5.2)

Go down two inches, pause slightly, go down two more inches.

Figure 5.1

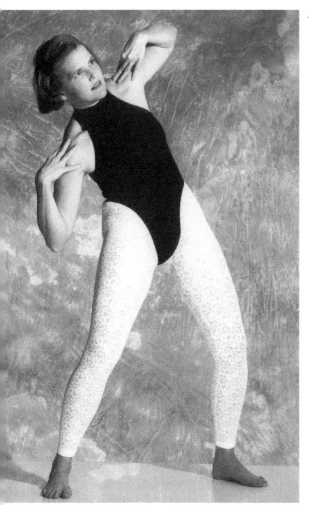

Figure 5.2 Push-up

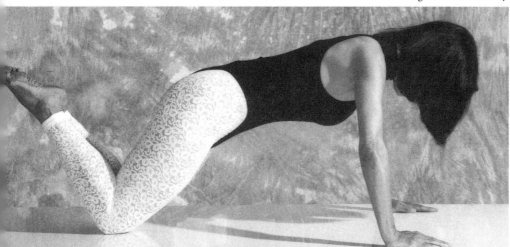

Then come up. The rhythm is down, down. Count. Then it's up, up. Always count on the second move down.

Try to do ten of these push-ups. If you can't do ten at first, do as many as possible and work up to ten by the end of the week.

If ten push-ups are relatively easy for you to do, add another set of ten. But remember, if you're a beginner, doing even five of these push-ups is great.

OUTSTRETCHED

Repeat the two stretches from last week. The first is: Hands to the floor and hold for a count of thirty. Keep your weight forward on the balls of your feet. Then, without moving your hips, take your right hand and reach to your left knee. This week, if you can, take hold of your calf instead of your knee and stretch your nose to your left knee. Keep your left arm extended overhead and behind you. Don't shift your weight. Keep it on the balls of your feet and hold for a count of thirty. Now move over to your right knee/calf and with your nose to this knee hold for a count of thirty with your right arm up and back. (Figure 5.3) Remember, if you have any problems with your back—do this stretch with both knees slightly bent.

You'll feel more flexible this week, so you can hold for the count of thirty with a little more ease. Continue to stretch throughout the thirty counts, loosening up as you hold.

The same advice goes for the straddle stretch on the floor. Where you were stiff last week you'll be somewhat more flexible this week, so getting into the stretch will be less difficult. You'll want to take advantage of those looser muscles to press into the stretch throughout the thirty counts. (Figure 5.4)

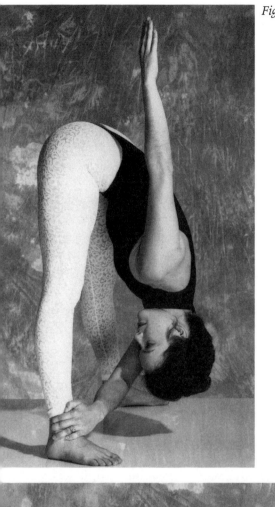

Figure 5.3

Figure 5.4

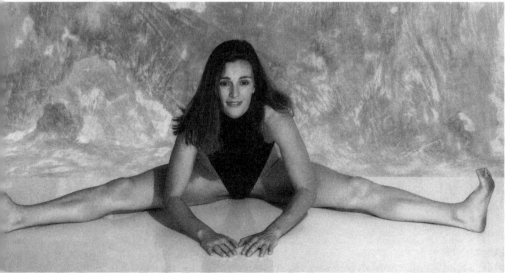

BACK AT THE BARRE

Let's start in First Position. Heels together, lifted one inch off the floor, suck in your tummy, tuck your pelvis, and bend your knees two inches.

Check your upper-body posture. Make sure you're lifted up—not hunched over. Start by rotating your shoulders up, back, and down. (Figure 5.5)

This week you'll add a third tuck at each of the three levels. So squeeze your seat and tuck, tuck, tuck. That's the rhythm. You loosen your squeeze between tucks but don't let go. Keep your bottom tucked under.

Now lower one inch and tuck, tuck, tuck. And go down to your third level and tuck, tuck, tuck. At this third level tuck *four* times and *hold* for a count of ten.

This week you're going to add a *sixth* repetition to complete one set. In other words, you do the tuck, tuck, tuck motion at all three levels (four tucks on the third level) six times.

For the second set of six repetitions you raise your right arm off the barre so your hand is above your head. This will help your posture and balance. You'll feel your upper body lifting and it will help you isolate the stretch in your quads. (Figure 5.6)

At some point you may want to give up. It's only natural. *Don't.* You can do it. We've seen the most out-of-shape women get past that "I can't" point, and once they do . . . they're in for the duration.

This is your time to exercise that control over your body. Have your mind talk to your body. You can do it.

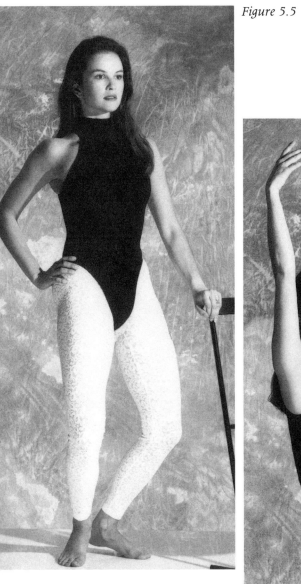

Figure 5.5

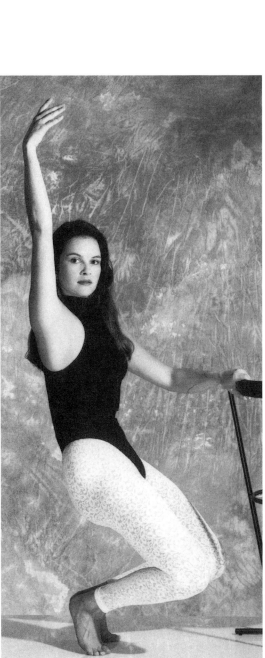

Figure 5.6

SECOND POSITION

Place your feet shoulder-width apart, with your heels one inch off the floor. Suck in your tummy, tuck your pelvis and bend your knees two inches. (Figure 5.7)

Just as you did in First Position, you're going to add a third tuck at each level and a sixth repetition in each set. So it goes like this: tuck, tuck, tuck . . . down an inch and tuck, tuck, tuck. Go down a third inch and tuck three times. On the third tuck, *hold* for a count of ten and then go back up to the first level, where your knees are bent two inches, and start the down/tucking motion again. Do the movement six times to complete the first set.

You'll be feeling this most in your quads and if your tuck is right the muscle will be working from the top of your quad—at the pubic bone—down to your knee.

Do a second set. Do not stop between sets. But do take the time to reaffirm your pelvic tuck and make sure your chest is lifted high, pulling up on your rib cage. Just imagine you have a string pulling you up straight and tall.

After you've completed your second set, it's time to stretch with legs apart and your hands on the floor. Hold for a count of thirty. While you're holding, be sure to pull up on the quads—don't just let them hang there. (See Figure 3.4, page 39)

Now move to your left leg with your nose pointing at your left knee and your right hand holding your left ankle. Your left arm is up in the air. Again, don't forget to pull up on the quad muscles by tightening your knees. Hold for a count of thirty and switch legs, repeating the motion and holding for thirty.

When you stand up from this position, be sure to bend your knees slightly before you lift your torso. That will lessen the load on your back.

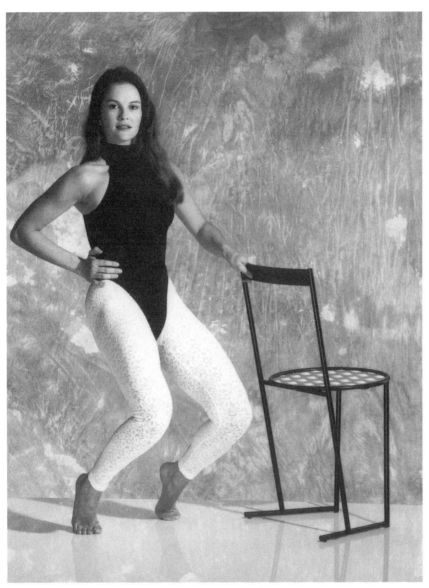

Figure 5.7

THIRD POSITION

This is a new position for us this week. Stand with your feet hip-width apart and turned out. Your knees and toes should be pointed out to the side with your knees lined up directly out over your toes. Bend your knees two inches. Lift your left heel up first and then lift your right heel up as high off the floor as you can. It's easier to lift one heel at a time and you'll have a better chance at balancing yourself than if you lifted both heels simultaneously. Be aware of your upper-body posture here. Make sure your chest is lifted, your shoulders squared and back. (Figure 5.8)

Be sure your heels stay high as you go through your repetitions.

Figure 5.8 Third Position

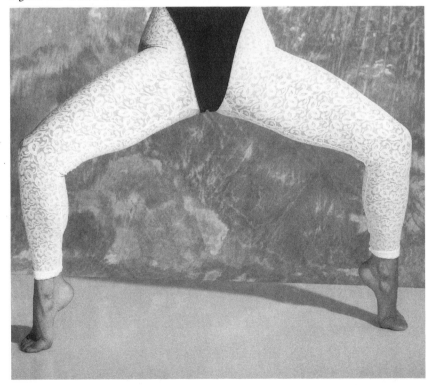

By shifting your weight onto your toes you'll bring the hamstrings and butt into play and take the pressure off the knees.

In this position, you do three tucks on three levels. So it goes like this: Tuck, tuck, tuck, lower one inch, and tuck, tuck, tuck. Lower another inch to the third level and tuck, tuck, tuck. That's a count of one. Now go back up to the first level and repeat three tucks at each level. Do a total of six repetitions to complete one set.

By now, your legs may be shaking. And you may be feeling a warm sensation. Good. You're doing everything right. Do a second set of six repetitions in the Third Position.

STRETCH IT OUT

It's time to stretch those quads by doing the Standing Quad Stretch you learned in the first week.(See Figure 4.2, page 45)

With your standing leg bent, bend your other knee and take your foot in your hand. Squeeze your butt hard and tilt your pelvis forward. You'll feel the upper half of your quad engaging in the stretch as you pull your bent leg back toward your seat. Remember, *don't* pull your heel into your seat. Keep it about three inches away.

Hold for a count of twenty and switch legs, repeating the stretch.

TO THE WALL

Take your ball with you and lie on the floor. This exercise is going to work your inner thighs (adductors). With your knees bent, put your feet up on the wall, and place the ball securely between your knees. Place your hips in line with your knees. Your knees should be perpendicular to the wall. Now squeeze your butt and rotate your pelvis up. *Hold.* (Figure 5.9)

Squeeze the ball by pushing your thighs together and hold for a count of three. Release the ball just enough to lessen the tension but not enough to drop the ball. Now squeeze again. Do this a total of thirty times to complete one set. Repeat the set.

Release the ball and hug your knees. Place the soles of your feet together and let your knees fall out to the side. Bring your feet in as close as you can while you stretch your inner thighs for a count of twenty. (Figure 5.10)

Put your feet back up against the wall. Keep them shoulder-width apart. This time, without the ball, squeeze your seat tightly. Slowly rotate your pelvis up, up, then down, down. You really work your

Figure 5.9

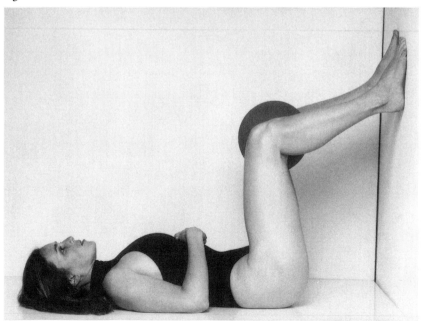

seat here if you squeeze tightly and move methodically. Do not lift your back off the floor. Count at the top. Do a total of thirty combinations of the up, up, down, down movement to complete one set. (Figure 5.11)

Now do a second set. Hug your knees to stretch it out.

Figure 5.10

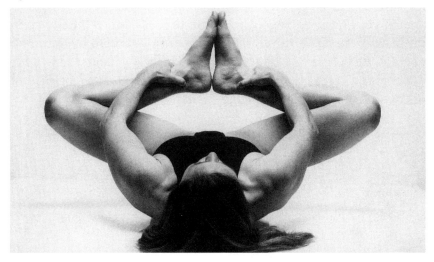

Figure 5.11

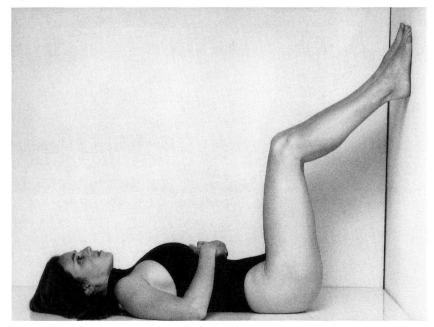

COOLING IT

It's time for the cool-down stretch. Move away from the wall. Lie flat on the floor with both knees bent. Lift your left leg and hold on to it with both hands. You should be looser this week, so try to reach for your calf or ankle and flex your foot. Now straighten the knee and lift your head up toward your kneecap. You'll feel the stretch in the back of the knee, through the hamstring and up to the insertion point at the base of the butt. Pull your leg back as close to the body as possible. This way you're elongating the muscle. Hold for a count of thirty and switch legs. (Figure 5.12)

Figure 5.12

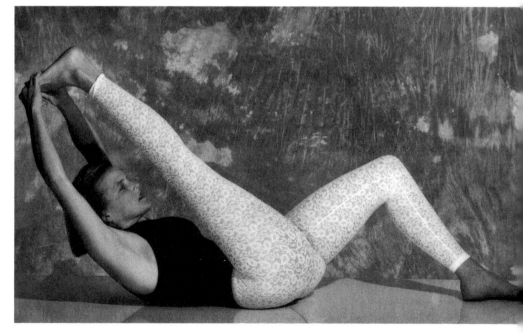

You should pat yourself on the back. You've completed the Week Two workout. Do the workout at least three times this week.

We know you're going to feel some stiffness as a result of this week's work. Don't worry about it. Revel in it. After all, that stiffness means you've been working your muscles—strengthening them and stretching them into shape.

In addition to shaping your muscles, there are other benefits to our exercises. They help prevent bone loss, since weight-bearing exercises like ours help build lean muscle tissue and bone mass. And these exercises help reduce the risk for diabetes since studies show every good workout can increase the ability of muscles to absorb insulin and to process sugar. And we take weak and popping knees and strengthen ligaments and tendons to make strong and happy knees.

Right now you should be feeling stronger and happier because you're ready to face week number three of our workout. You're on your way toward World Class Legs.

CHAPTER SIX

WEEK THREE

By now you should be feeling much more limber. One of the by-products of our workout is that from the tilting of the pelvis and the stretches that we do, you're developing a more flexible and healthier spine. Every time you tuck and with every stretch you do, you're taking the pressure off your lower back and expanding your range of motion.

At this point you must be noticing that you're less stiff in the morning when you get out of bed. Your walk is a little looser and we bet you're even starting to feel more attractive as a result. Well, let's press on. The best is yet to come.

This week's warm-up is the same as last week's but we're adding Triceps Push-ups to work the back of the arm. You know the area we're talking about. Wave your arm in the air, then stop. Where the skin keeps flapping—that's your triceps and it's traditionally one of the weakest spots on a woman's body.

Go ahead and put on your music and start your warm-up.

- Sixty Leg Lifts with your legs alternately raised toward hands extended forward from your shoulders

- Continue the leg lifting sixty times while your arms reach out to the side and up and down

· Hands on your shoulders, pelvic tuck, knees bent. Bend sideways—with your elbow pointed to the floor—come up and bend to the other side and back up to the center. Do this twenty times.

Now you're at your first set of push-ups, on your hands and knees, stomach pulled in and your hands facing forward. Try to increase the number of push-ups by at least five by the end of the week. Add one the first day, three the second, and by the third workout this week, try adding five. However, don't feel discouraged if you can't get up to ten or more. Do the best you can.

After you've completed your first set of push-ups, change the position of your hands by turning your fingers in about forty-five degrees toward each other. Keep your hands shoulder-width apart—any closer would make these next push-ups too hard to do. And don't forget to keep your knees bent. (Figure 6.1)

A reminder: It's very important to keep your abdominals pulled in with your pelvis tucked. That will protect your back from injury.

Shift your weight onto your arms and lower two inches, then two more inches. Count at the bottom. So it goes like this: down, down . . . one. Up, up. Down, down . . . two. Up, up. Try for ten of these triceps push-ups. If you can't do ten, do as many as you can.

Figure 6.1

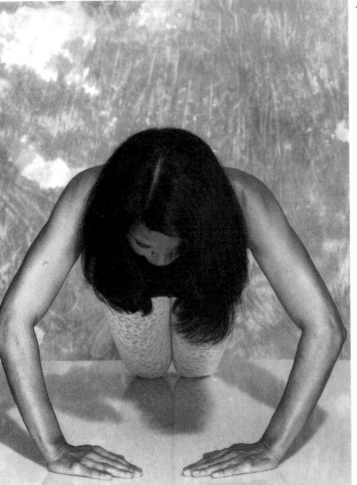

MARK YOUR STRETCH

We're adding a new stretch here, for the arm muscles you just worked. Take your right arm and raise it straight up over your head. Now bend your elbow and move your hand behind you so it touches your shoulder blade. It should look as if you're trying to pat yourself on the back.

Take your left arm and reach it up over your head. Take hold of your right elbow with your left hand and gently press that right elbow back and down, reaching your right hand as low down on your back as you can to maximize the stretch. You'll feel the stretch in your triceps. Hold for a count of ten. (Figure 6.2)

Release that hold and take your right arm around in front of you—across your chest. Use your left hand to take hold of your elbow and gently pull it across you. You'll feel the stretch in both the biceps and the triceps. Hold it here for a count of ten.

Release the stretch and switch arms, reaching up and back with your left arm and holding your left elbow with your right hand, gently pressing it back and down on your shoulder blade. Hold for a count of ten, then release your arm and bring it across your chest. Hold your left elbow with your right hand for a count of ten and release.

Now it's back to the two basic stretches we started with in Week One. (See Figures 3.4 and 3.5, page 39) First, hands to the floor and hold for thirty. If you've had any trouble the first two weeks getting your hands flat on the floor, the turning point may be this week. You're developing flexibility that will allow you to get in and out of our stretches more easily, and throughout the count of thirty you'll feel your muscles elongating. Always pull up on the thigh muscles and hold them in a flexed position throughout the count. You should be able to see your muscles contracting and gaining definition.

After you've touched your nose to each knee and completed those stretches, get on the floor for the Straddle Stretch. (Figure 3.6, page 39) Keep your legs as far apart as possible and bring your torso down between your legs, reaching your hands out farther than you did last week. By the end of this week, you may be able to get your hands parallel to your lower calves. Feel your spine stretch. Now move your hands over to your left leg and place your arms on both sides of your leg, straddling your leg with your arms. Hold the stretch for a count of thirty—stretching farther throughout the count. Gently—no jarring or quick motions—move your hands over to your right side and place your arms on either side of that leg. Hold the count for thirty.

It's time to get up and go over to your barre. Rise slowly and keep your knees bent—that will take pressure off your lower back as you move.

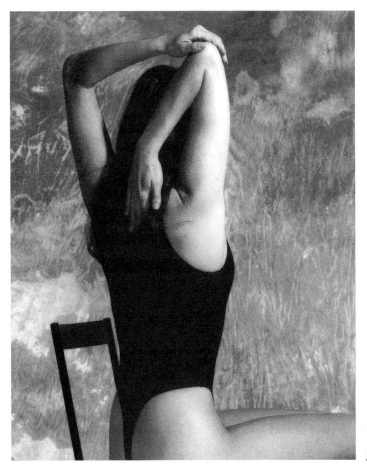

Figure 6.2

SHIFTING INTO FIRST

Start in First Position with your right hand on the barre, heels touching and lifted one inch off the floor. Bend your knees two inches and lift your left arm overhead for balance. Don't raise your shoulders. Keep them back and down. (Figure 6.3)

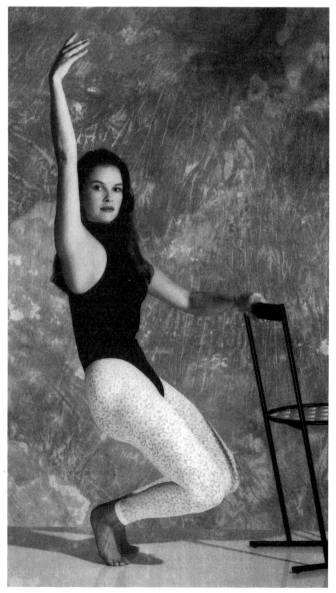

Figure 6.3
Shifting into
First

Now, tuck, release. Remember, the release is minimal. Don't let go completely, just a little and then go right back into a tight squeeze. We're adding a tuck at each level here, to bring the count to four.

After you've tucked four times, drop an inch by bending your knees and tuck four times on the second level. Drop a third inch and tuck four times and *hold* for a count of ten. Hold tight. Don't let go. Feel the stretch in your quads. The harder you squeeze your butt, the more strength you'll get, making this movement easier and more effective.

Repeat the down/tuck movement with the hold six times to complete one set.

Do the Standing Quad Stretch: Standing with your right knee bent and your left foot in your left hand, tuck your pelvis and stretch back your left quad. The bigger the tuck, the more elongated the stretch. If you feel cramping in your hamstring you're not tucking enough. Hold the stretch for a count of twenty. Turn and switch legs. Hold the right quad stretch for a count of twenty. (See Figure 4.2, page 45)

Move back into First Position, this time holding the barre with your left hand and raising your right arm overhead. Check your posture in the mirror. Do a second set of six repetitions, tucking four times at each of the three levels and *hold* at the bottom level of each repetition for a count of ten.

Repeat the standing Quad Stretch. This time the pull on the front of your thighs will feel a little less intense since you've been stretching out your quads as you go.

SECOND POSITION

With your feet shoulder-width apart, raise your heels one inch off the floor. Suck in your tummy, squeeze your butt, and tuck your pelvis. Bend your knees two inches. Raise your right arm overhead

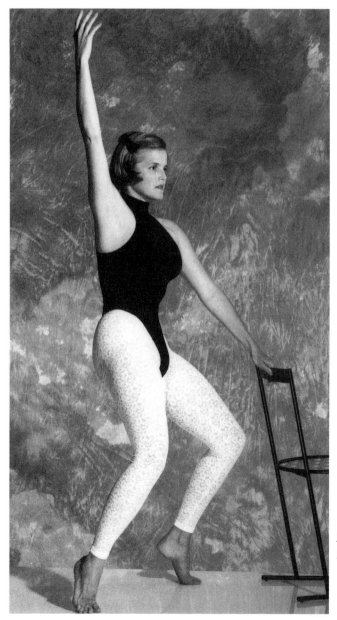

Figure 6.4
Second Position

while you hold your barre with your left hand. This will keep your chest high and your shoulders back. (Figure 6.4)

This time you're going to tuck four times at each of the three levels. It goes like this: Tuck, tuck, tuck, tuck, lower an inch to level two and tuck, tuck, tuck, tuck. Lower a third inch and tuck, tuck, tuck, tuck. That's a count of one. Rise back up to the first level, where your knees are bent two inches, and start tucking again. Do this tuck/down movement six times to complete one set.

Without stopping, keep your right arm raised and do six more repetitions. Your quads are going to feel tight. Remember, squeeze your butt, it will help. If your legs shake, it's OK—it means your muscles are working hard and that's exactly what we want them to be doing.

If you need a drink of water about now, stop and take it. You don't have to worry about missing a beat with our workout. You can pick up at any time. Just keep the music going.

THIRD POSITION

Stand at the barre with your legs turned out wide. Your knees should be pointed out to the side, straight out over your toes. Bend your knees two inches out over your toes. Lift your left heel and

Figure 6.5 Third Position

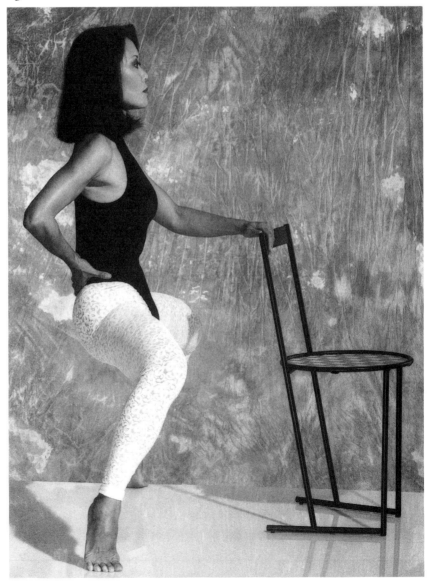

then your right heel up off the floor as high as you can. Shift your weight onto your toes as much as possible. That will ensure that you work your hamstrings and take the pressure off your knees. (Figure 6.5)

Now tuck four times, then lower one inch by bending your knees and tuck four times at this second level. Lower one more inch and tuck four times at this third level. That's a count of one. Go back up to the first level, where your knees are bent two inches, and repeat the four tucks at each of the three levels. Do a total of six repetitions to complete one set.

Do the Standing Quad Stretch. Bend your right knee—this is your standing leg. Bend your left knee and lift your left foot behind you. Hold it in your left hand. Squeeze your seat and tuck your pelvis. Feel your left quad stretching? Elongate the stretch by deepening your tuck. Suck in that stomach. Hold for a count of twenty. Now do the same, lifting your right foot.

If you're feeling strong enough, do a second set in Third Position. Repeat the same action as above: four tucks at each of the three levels. Do it six times to complete a second set. If you do a second set, don't forget to finish with the Standing Quad Stretch.

USING THE WALL

Move over to the wall and lie down, back flat on the floor. Put your feet flat against the wall with your knees bent and your seat directly under your knees.

Place the ball between your knees. Now tuck your pelvis and use your thighs to squeeze the ball. Squeeze the ball twice, then tuck your pelvis while you're squeezing the ball. Do *not* lift your back off the floor—only your seat tucks up. The movement goes like this: In, in, up. Count one. Repeat the motion methodically. Do it thirty times to complete one set. (Figure 6.6)

Keep the thighs squeezing and keep the seat squeezing—even on the release of the seat between counts. After you've done a complete set, start a second set and repeat the in, in, up motion another thirty times.

This exercise is great for working your butt, inner thighs, and outer thighs.

STICK TO THE WALL

Keep the same position at the wall, but put the ball aside for now. Your feet stay shoulder-width apart. Tuck your pelvis and tilt it up and then up again. Count one. Slowly and methodically take it down and down again to the starting position. The trick is not to release your tuck when you're back down. Stay squeezing and lift again. Lift only your seat off the floor by squeezing your butt. Don't lift your back. Your lower back presses into the floor. Do this up, up, down, down movement thirty times to complete one set. Then go right into a second set of thirty. (Figure 6.7)

Now hug your knees. That will help stretch out your butt. You can stretch your inner thighs here by putting the soles of your feet together and opening out your knees. Hold your feet in as close to your seat as you can. (Figure 5.10, page 67) That should really feel good right now. Do each of these stretches for at least a count of twenty before you move on.

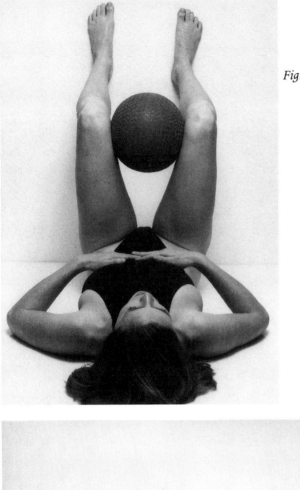

Figure 6.6

Figure 6.7

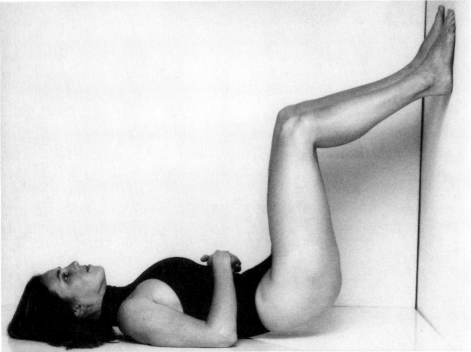
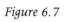

THE UP SIDE

We're about to give you a leg up on your trip toward World Class Legs. You're going to do leg lifts combined with the pelvic tuck that will work the sides of your thighs and butt more quickly than any traditional leg lift.

Lie on your right side fully extended with your left leg on top of your right. Put your head on your right arm and plant your left elbow firmly in front of you. Keep your elbow in that position throughout this entire section. It will keep you from injuring your lower back and will anchor you in front. You don't want to tilt back at all. (Figure 6.8)

Now squeeze your seat. Lock those gluteus muscles together. Keep this contraction at all times. Keeping your left leg straight with your knee pointed forward, lift it up two inches and down two inches. Never touch your heels. Never lose that tuck.

You're going to do fifty leg lifts in this position. If, at any time, you

Figure 6.8

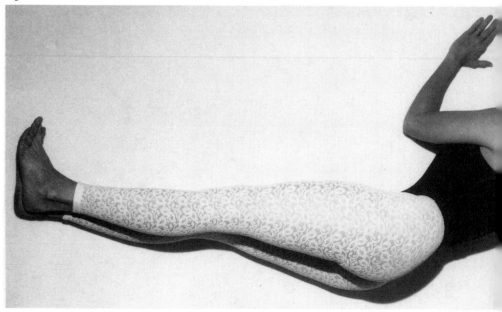

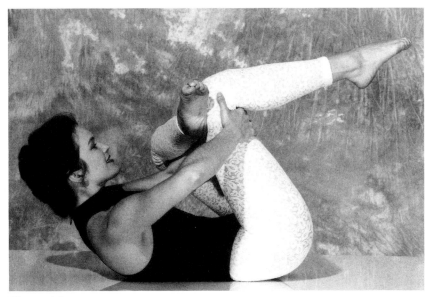

Figure 6.9

feel yourself slipping out of your tuck, stop and reaffirm the tuck. You can do leg lifts all you want, but unless you're squeezing your butt you won't be molding it.

After you've completed fifty lifts with your left leg, lie on your back and stretch out your left leg by crossing your left ankle over your right knee. To do this, keep your right leg up in the air while you cross your ankle over the top of your knee. Reach around and pull your right leg as close to your torso as possible. You'll feel the pull along the outside of your left thigh. At the same time you'll be stretching out the hamstrings of your right leg and your butt. Hold for a count of twenty. (Figure 6.9)

Switch legs. Lie on your left side with your right leg on top of your left. Make sure your knee is pointed forward. Plant that right elbow firmly in front of you. Now squeeze that butt as hard as you can and lock in that tuck. Lift your right leg up two inches and lower it two inches. Again, never let your heels touch and make sure your knee doesn't bend. Do fifty lifts with your right leg.

*   *   *

Stretch out your right leg by lying on your back and lifting your left leg up in the air. Now take your right ankle and cross it over your left knee. Reach around with your hands and pull your left leg as close to your torso as is comfortable. You'll feel the stretch in your right outer thigh, your left hamstring, and your butt.

To make sure you're getting your outer thigh/hip area and butt into shape, we've got one more set of leg lifts for you to do this week.

Lie on your right side, your head on your extended right arm and your left elbow planted firmly in front of you. Bring your legs out in front of you at a ninety-degree angle to your torso. Squeeze your butt and tuck. Lock in that tuck. Raise your top leg in two moves, making sure it doesn't go any higher than your hip. If your tuck is a good, strong one, you won't be able to lift higher than hip level. So the motion is up, up, down, down. Count at the top. Do fifty of these leg lifts. (Figure 6.10)

Figure 6.10

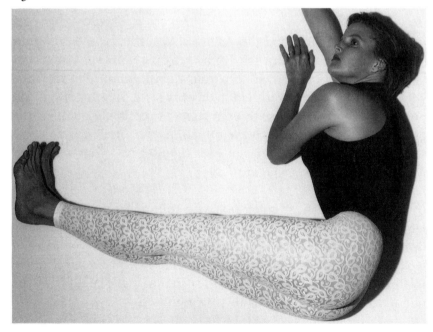

Move over to your back and stretch out your left leg by crossing your left ankle over your right knee which is bent. Hold for a count of twenty.

Switch sides. Lie on your left side so your right leg is on top. Move your legs out in front of you so they're at a right angle to your torso. Make sure your right elbow is firmly planted in front of you and keep it there. Now tuck and lock it in. Lift up, up, and count. Lower down, down. Don't lift any higher than hip level. If your leg goes higher than hip level, you're not holding a good enough tuck, so stop and reaffirm. Then go on to complete fifty lifts with your right leg.

It's time to stretch it out. Cross your right ankle over your bent left knee. Reach out and pull that left leg as close to your torso as you can and hold it for a count of twenty.

Great work! Let's move on to the Cool-down Stretch.

COOL IT

Stay right there on the floor, lying on your back with both legs bent at the knee, feet flat on the floor. Lift your left leg and reach for the leg with both hands. By now you should be flexible enough to reach for your calf or even your ankle. Pull your leg as close to your body as you can. (See Figure 5.12, page 68)

Keep your stomach pulled in. Flex your foot and straighten your knee. Lift your head up toward the knee. You'll feel the stretch from the back of your knee up your hamstring and through your butt. Hold that stretch for a count of thirty. Then switch legs and repeat the stretch with your right leg. Hold it for a count of thirty.

Well, you did it! Once you get through this third week you can feel very accomplished. Lots of people don't make it this far. But then you're not lots of people. You're a contender for World Class Legs!

CHAPTER SEVEN

WEEK FOUR

We hope that by this week you're starting to get excited about the way you look and feel. Regardless of what else is going on in your life, your health is one place where, by now, you're proving you can take control. And once you do, you'll find that you can run the rest of your life a lot better, too.

The women who come into our studio to work out all have busy schedules but know they can operate more effectively elsewhere if they devote these workout hours to themselves. The discipline spills over into other work. The dividends pay off in all areas of their lives.

Let's face it, life can be frustrating. Some days it feels like everything's going wrong. But you've got something to look forward to. When you pick up your heels and squeeze your butt, you're squeezing out those frustrations. And at the same time you're improving the way you look. You're shaping a better attitude while you're shaping a better body.

Now take a deep breath. This is your time. Let's tuck away those worries, squeeze out those disappointments, and build a cadre of admirers along with your own self-confidence and your World Class Legs.

GET YOUR HEART INTO IT

We hope you've been keeping up your thirty-minute cardiovascular routine either on alternate days or along with our workout. But even if you go right to our warm-up routine, be sure you're getting your pulse rate into your target heart range (see chapter 3 for chart). There's a by-product to this level of exertion. With vigorous exercise, your brain releases endorphins, which are our bodies' own version of painkillers. Endorphins control your body's response to stress, and many athletes report endorphins give them a natural high. So utilize what nature's offered. Turn on that music, get that heart rate up, those endorphins flowing, and lift your spirits as you lift your legs.

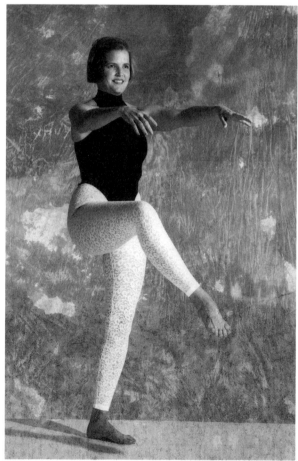

Figure 7.1

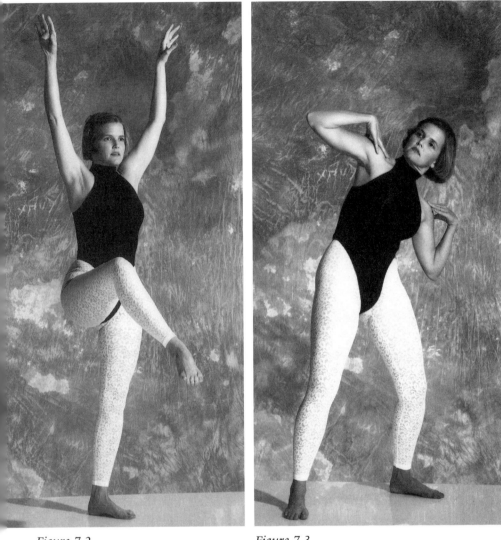

Figure 7.2   Figure 7.3

Stick to the same basic warm-up this week. Sixty leg lifts, raising your legs up to your arms which are extended forward from your shoulders. (Figure 7.1)

Next, move your arms out to the side, and up and down while you continue to lift your legs another sixty times—thirty lifts of each leg. (Figure 7.2)

Now stop and plant your feet firmly on the floor. Place your hands on your shoulders, tuck your pelvis, bend your knees and bend your body to the side, back to center, and to the other side. Each side, center, side is a count of one. Do twenty of these. (Figure 7.3)

Move down to the floor for push-ups: on your knees, with your hands forward on the floor, shoulder-width apart, pelvis tucked, and tummy in. Go down two inches, down again two inches, and count one. Now rise back up and then up again. Repeat for a count of ten to complete one set. At the start of this week you should be doing at least ten push-ups. And by the end of the week you'll be completing a second set of ten.

Breathe deeply. Inhale when you're at the top, starting the push-up. Then exhale when you're making the most effort, when you're at the bottom ready to push up.

After you've completed two sets of regular push-ups, turn your hands in toward each other. (See Figure 6.1, page 73) Check to make sure your tummy's pulled in and start your triceps push-ups. Lower two inches and then again two inches. Your chest should touch the tops of your hands. Then push up two inches and again two more inches. Optimally, you worked up to ten of these triceps push-ups last week. If you did, try to do another ten this week.

STRETCHING TIME

Take this time to stretch, starting with your arms. Raise your right arm up, bend it back at the elbow, and reach down behind you—as if to pat yourself on the back. With your left hand reach up over your head and push down—gently—on your right elbow. (See Figure 6.2, page 75) You'll feel this stretch in the back of your arms. Hold it for a count of ten. Release and switch arms and stretch your left arm.

Stretch slowly to avoid injury. This way you'll feel your safety zone, and won't stretch so fast and far that you tear a muscle. Pulled muscles come from quick starts and stops.

For your next stretch, your legs are apart and you bend forward placing your hands on the floor. Hold for a count of thirty. During that time your muscles will loosen and your stretch will get deeper. Now, with your nose pointed to your left knee and your right hand on your left ankle—your left arm is extended above you—hold that stretch for a count of thirty. Remember to suck in your stomach and pull up on your quads. Here again you'll feel the stretch get deeper as you hold through the count. (Figure 7.4)

Figure 7.4

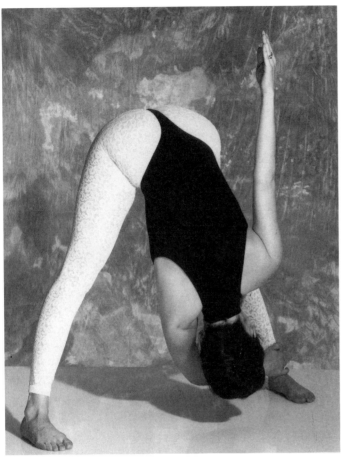

Now move over to your right knee and place your left hand on your right ankle. Your right arm is extended above you. Hold for thirty and throughout that count you'll feel your spine and your hamstrings getting more flexible.

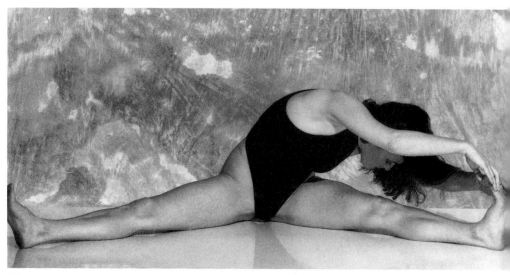

Figure 7.5

Next, sit on the floor with your legs spread wide. Make sure your legs are down, flat against the floor, and your toes are pointed up. Slowly bend forward, placing your torso between your legs and extending your arms as far as you can. Don't force this, but as you count to thirty, try to gently flex farther and farther forward. Then move around to your left leg and place your upper body over that leg. Keep your arms on either side of the leg and if you can, grab hold of your foot and pull yourself flat against your leg. Hold for a count of thirty and move over to your right leg and repeat for a count of thirty. (Figure 7.5)

First Position:

Let's start our barre work in First Position with your heels touching, lifted one inch off the floor. Hold on to the barre with your left hand. Suck in your tummy and tuck your pelvis; bring your knees to starting position, bent two inches. Check your posture and lift your right arm up over your head. That will help you balance so your bottom half is doing all the work.

You're going to tuck four times at the first level. Tuck and release but don't release far—keep those hips forward—and tuck, release, tuck, release, tuck, release. Bend your knees another inch and tuck four times. Bend another inch and tuck four times. We're going to add something new at this point.

After you tuck four times at the bottom level, instead of holding for a count of ten you'll plié (*plee-ay*) ten times. (See Figure 6.3, page 76)

The plié is a small ballet movement. Your legs are bent and your back is held straight and you move down an inch and up an inch. Don't travel any more than one inch each way. Do not bounce—move smoothly down and up ten times. Then go back to the starting position, where your knees are bent two inches, and tuck four times again to start your second repetition.

You'll be doing six repetitions and at the bottom level of each repetition you'll do the ten pliés. After you've completed the first set, take a moment to check yourself in the mirror. There's a natural tendency here to bend over. Be aware of this and make sure you straighten up. Then move on to a second set of six repetitions with four tucks at each of the three levels and again the ten pliés at the bottom of each repetition. Your legs may shake because you're pushing hard on this one. But don't worry, they're getting stronger.

It's time to stretch them out with a new quad stretch. Make sure you're on the carpet or a pad because you'll need to protect your knees.

On the floor, put your weight on your left knee and extend your right leg forward. Bend it at the knee and point your toes straight ahead. Now put your chest down on to your right knee and slide

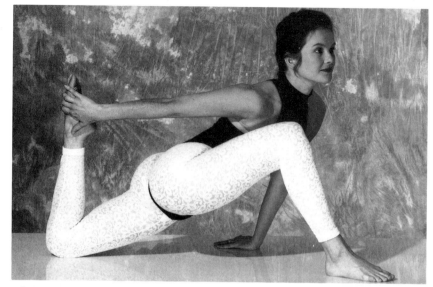

Figure 7.6

your left knee back. Press your left hip forward and down. Lift your left foot and reach back around with your right hand and hold it for a count of ten. (Figure 7.6) You'll really feel the stretch in the quad and this stretch will open up your hip area, too. That's especially good for those of you who sit all day. You tend to get tight in the hip area. This will loosen you up.

After you hold for a count of ten, switch legs and repeat, this time putting your weight on your right knee and moving your left leg forward—bent at the knee with toes pointing straight ahead. Now put your chest down on to your knee and slide your right knee back. Press your right hip forward and down. Lift your right foot and reach back with your left hand and hold it for a count of ten. Feel your quad stretching out? It should feel pretty good about now.

Second Position

Move into Second Position. Your feet are shoulder-width apart. Lift your heels one inch off the floor. Suck in your tummy and tuck your pelvis. Bend your knees two inches. Check your posture. Lift your chest up so it feels like it's lifting off your rib cage. Now start your tucking. Do four tucks at the first level, four tucks at the second level, and four at the third level. Now, hold it, because we've got a new movement for you here.

At the third level down, circle your hips five times to the right and then five times to the left. Then lift back up to the first level and start your second repetition, tucking four times at level one; bend your knees one inch and tuck four times at level two; and then bend one more inch and tuck four more times. Once again, circle your hips five times to the right and five times to the left while you're down at the third level. (Figure 7.7)

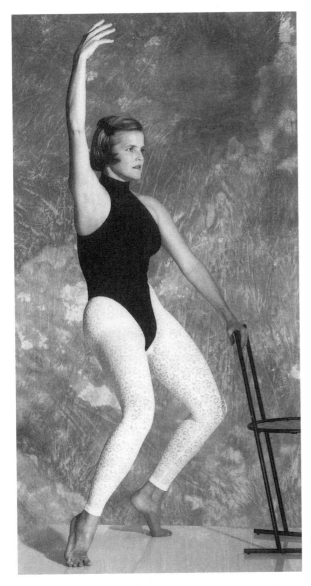

Figure 7.7

Do six of these repetitions to complete one set. Do two sets. Then go back down to the floor and finish up with the quad stretch.

Put your weight on your left knee and move your right leg forward—bending it at the knee. Your toes should point straight ahead. Lean your chest against your right leg and slide your left knee back. Press your left hip forward and down. Reach behind you with your right hand and lift your left foot, pulling it toward your seat. Hold this stretch for a count of ten and switch legs, repeating the stretch on your right leg.

Shift into Third

This week you're going to work the Third Position with the ball. Instead of standing with your legs turned out, stand with your legs parallel and apart. Put the ball between your knees, holding your legs close enough to keep the ball securely in place. Your knees and toes should be pointed forward. Bend your knees two inches. Now tuck four times. Lower an inch, and keep squeezing so the ball stays secure. Repeat the four tucks at the second level and then again on the third level down. Do six repetitions of this tuck with the ball to complete one set. Do two of these sets. (Figure 7.8)

Here we have a new move for you. Stay in Third Position with the ball between your knees and, starting with your knees bent two inches, lower another two inches and scoop your hips forward. The scoop is an exaggerated tuck. Keep the tuck as you come up and then lower and scoop again. Your moves should be slow, smooth, and continuous. Do eight repetitions to complete one set. (Figure 7.9)

To stretch out your quads, put your weight on your left knee and move your right leg forward, bending it at the knee. Your toes point forward. Rest your chest against your right leg and slide your left knee back. Press your left hip forward and down and then reach behind you with your right hand and pull your left foot closer to your seat. Hold for a count of ten. (See Figure 7.6, page 96)

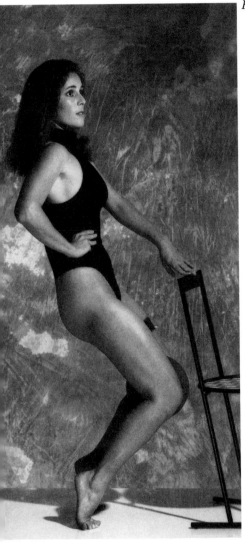

Figure 7.8

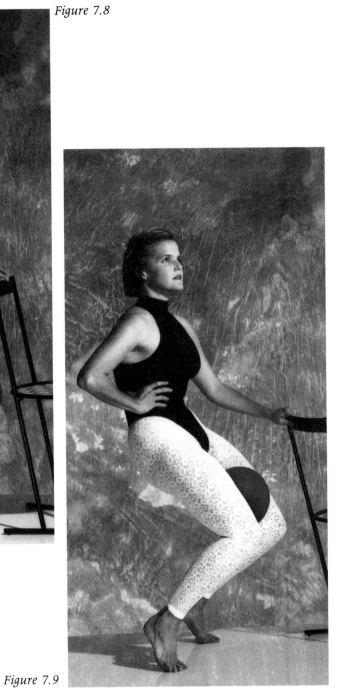

Figure 7.9

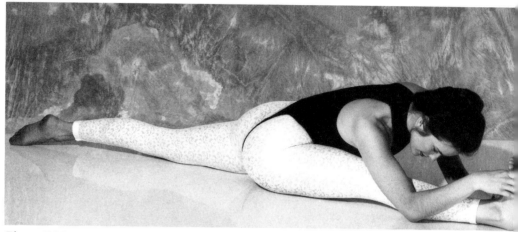

Figure 7.10

As you lower your left foot to the floor, extend your left leg farther back and your right leg forward until it's straight out in front of you. Your elbows are bent slightly on either side of your right leg. Put your nose to your knee and hold for a count of ten. (Figure 7.10) This will really stretch your hamstrings. Be careful never to bounce this stretch. Move into it slowly and hold it steadily. Your flexibility will increase over the next weeks and you'll be able to go farther down into more of a front split. But even if you never make it down into a true split, this stretch will work your hamstrings all the way up to your butt.

After you hold for a count of ten, switch legs so that your right foot is back and your left leg is forward. Repeat the quad stretch by holding your right foot behind you for a count of ten. Then move into the hamstring stretch by extending your right leg farther back and straightening your left leg and extending it. Keep your elbows bent slightly and put your nose to your knee and hold for a count of ten.

HAVE A BALL

With the ball between your knees, lie with your feet flat against the
wall and your knees bent so that your hips are directly underneath
them. Squeeze your seat up and squeeze the ball. Hold for a count
of three. Release the ball slightly, then squeeze the ball again for a
count of three. Do this fifteen times, making sure you don't release
your seat. Keep it tilted up and squeezing hard. (Figure 7.11) Then
squeeze the ball in, in again, and tilt up. This in, in, up motion
counts as one. Do it fifteen times to complete a set. On the last
count, squeeze and hold for a count of ten. Then do two more sets
of fifteen—both times holding the last squeeze and tilt up for a count
of ten.

Figure 7.11

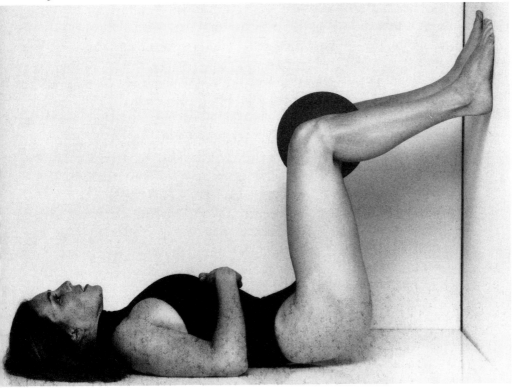

Now, without the ball, keep your feet and knees shoulder-width apart and tuck: Up, up, down, down, curling your lower spine up as you go but never lifting your back off the floor. Do twenty cycles of this up, up, down, down motion to complete one set. On the last up, squeeze your seat and hold your tuck for a count of ten. Release it and repeat the set. When you're done, hug your knees to your chest and stretch.

ON THE SIDE

Move away from the wall and lie on your right side on the floor. Extend your right arm and rest your head on this arm. Plant your left arm firmly on the floor in front of you. Now tuck your pelvis. Lock it into place. Lift your left leg up, up, then reverse: lower, lower. Do not lift it any higher than hip height and when you bring it down, do not touch your heels or rest your leg. It should stay in constant and steady motion: up, up, down, down. Do this fifty times. Make sure your knee is pointed straight ahead toward the mirror. On the last lift, hold—with your knee turned upward—for a count of ten. Don't fall back; it will put pressure on your lower back and negate the work. Be sure you're keeping your pelvic tuck. It's your insurance for a rounded butt.

Now, stretch your left outer thigh and butt by lying on your back and crossing your left ankle over your right knee which is extended in the air. Pull your right leg in as close as you can to maximize the stretch. Always keep your stomach in—don't let it pop out. Hold for a count of ten and switch legs, stretching your butt and right outer thigh by crossing your right ankle over your left knee. Hold for a count of ten.

It's time to work the right leg. Lie back on the floor—this time on your left side. Extend your left arm and rest your head on your arm. Plant your right arm firmly on the floor in front of you and tuck your pelvis. Lock in that tuck and lift your right leg up, up, then reverse: lower, lower. Remember, don't lift any higher than hip height and don't touch your heels or rest your leg when you lower it. Keep your motion constant and steady. It's up, up; down, down fifty times. On the last lift hold—making sure your knee is pointed straight ahead toward the mirror. Hold your last lift—with your knee turned upward—for a count of ten.

Let's stretch your right outer thigh and your butt by lying on your back and crossing your right ankle over your left knee which is extended in the air. Pull your left leg in close as you hold for a count of ten and switch legs, repeating the stretch for your left outer thigh and your butt.

Now go back to lying on your right side. This time, extend both your legs so they're in front of you at a ninety-degree angle to your torso. Your left leg is on top. Rotate your pelvis. Squeeze your seat. Lock your knees out straight and lift one inch, then lower one inch. You shouldn't lift any higher than hip height. If you're working properly with your pelvis tucked, you shouldn't be able to, anyway. Do this motion ten times. Pause. Now move your top leg one inch forward and one inch back. Do this ten times and pause. Now combine the two movements so it's one inch up and down to center and one inch forward and back to center—in an **L** shape. Repeat this combination ten times to complete a set. (Figure 7.12) Then repeat the set.

After you've worked your left leg, move over to your left side, lying with your right leg on top and both your legs extended out in

Figure 7.12

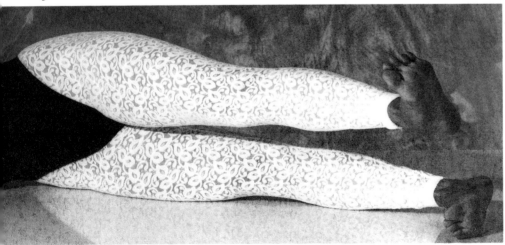

a ninety-degree angle to your torso. Repeat the moves you just did with your left leg. First lift then lower your right leg one inch up and one inch down. Do this ten times. Remember, keep your pelvis locked in that tuck. Move your right leg one inch forward and one inch back. Do this ten times and pause. Follow by combining the two movements so it's one inch up and down to center and one inch forward and back to center—in an L shape. Repeat this combination ten times to complete a set.

COOLING-OFF PERIOD

Lie on your back with both legs bent at the knee, feet flat on the floor. Lift your left leg and reach for it with both hands. (Figure 7.13)

Reach as high as you can. This week you may be able to grab your ankle or even your foot. Pull your leg as close to your body as possible. Don't let your tummy pop out. Suck it in while you flex your foot and straighten your knee. Lift your head toward the knee. You'll feel the stretch from the back of the knee all the way up to the

Figure 7.13

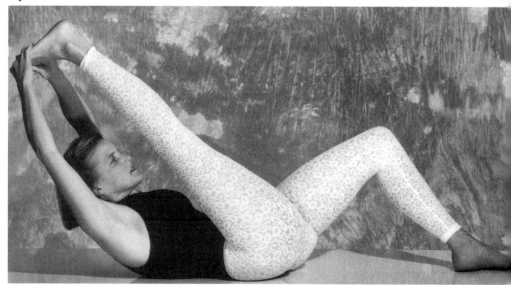

base of your butt. Hold for a count of thirty. Release and switch. Stretch your right leg. Hold for a count of thirty. Release and applaud.

You deserve applause for completing your fourth week. This may be tough work but it's a testimony to your spirit that you've made it through. You've now got more than a leg up in this quest for World Class Legs. You've got two legs up. And they're looking lean and mean. Keep going . . . you're shaping a longer, prettier future.

CHAPTER EIGHT

WEEK FIVE

THE SECRET INGREDIENT

You're about to turn a corner. Once you've made it this far, there's no turning back. You know how good it feels to take charge of your body. You know how much better your body looks and feels. You're trading in that slower, less fit version of you for a leaner, more efficient model and, boy, does that feel great. Those shapely new legs of yours are going to carry you through the next two weeks and then into a permanent program for World Class Legs. You've learned the secret ingredient. It's *you*!

You've decided you want to look good more than you want to eat that cream pie. Where you once got momentary pleasure from chewing a chocolate candy bar, you're now getting longer-lasting pleasure from stretching your muscles. Where you once had excuses for not exercising, you wouldn't dream of copping out now. We've seen it happen over and over again. World Class Legs will bring you a World Class Attitude.

So turn on the music—this would be a good week to start using the Pointer Sisters' "I'm So Excited." Now let's lift those legs as high as your spirits.

THE WARM-UP

We'll start with our (by now familiar) basic warm-up. Extend your arms in front of you at shoulder level and alternately lift your legs, reaching your toes toward your fingers. Do sixty of these leg lifts—alternating thirty right, thirty left.

Keep moving your legs and start moving your arms, pumping that heart good and strong. Move your arms out to the side—at shoulder level—and then lift them up and bring them back down to shoulder level. Do another sixty of the leg lifts while your arms pump up and down.

Now let's get your upper body into the act. Plant your feet. Put your hands on your shoulders and tuck your pelvis. Make sure your knees are bent and, with your arms, bend sideways, back up to center, and down to the other side so your elbows point down toward the floor. Each move of side, center, side is a count of one. Repeat the move twenty times.

PUSHING IT

Get down on the floor for push-ups. We're adding more again this week. On your knees, with your hands on the floor shoulder-width apart, pelvis tucked, and tummy in, go down two inches, down again two inches, and count one. Now rise up partway and then up again. Repeat for a count of twelve to complete one set. By the end of this week you'll be completing a second set of twelve. If you can do two sets right away—go for it. If not, add four push-ups each day until you complete two sets of twelve each.

After you've completed two sets of regular push-ups, turn your hands in toward each other. Check to make sure your tummy's pulled in and start your triceps push-ups. Lower two inches and then again two inches. Your chest should be grazing the top of your hands at the bottom, just before you push up two inches and again two more inches. Remember, each down, down, up, up is a count of one and you count at the bottom. Do twelve of these triceps push-ups to complete one set. Work up to two complete sets by the end of this fifth week.

STRETCHING FOR SUCCESS

All our stretches will ensure that your muscles get the maximum benefits from our strengthening exercises. Your first stretch of the day comes directly after the push-ups. You just worked on building your biceps and your triceps; now you want to stretch them out.

So, raise your right arm, extending it up over your head and then bend it back at the elbow. With your left hand, reach up and over your head to your right elbow. Then, gently push your right elbow back and down until you feel the stretch in the back of your arm. Hold for a count of twenty, increasing the stretch as you hold. (See Figure 6.2, page 75)

Now extend your right arm around in front of you, reaching toward your left shoulder. Use your left hand to grab your right elbow and pull it closer to your chest. Feel the stretch in your upper arm? Hold it for a count of twenty. (Figure 8.1)

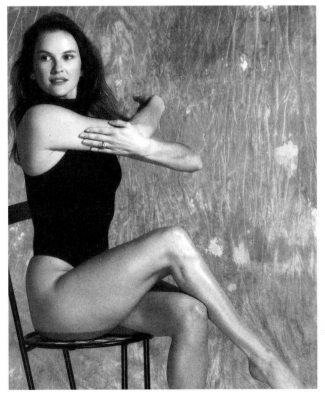

Figure 8.1

Switch arms and repeat both movements with your left arm. First bend it back behind you and use your right hand to gently push back and down on your elbow. Hold for a count of twenty, then reach your left arm around in front of you, extending your left hand past your right arm toward your back as you pull it closer to your chest with your right hand. Hold this stretch for a count of twenty.

Now let's stretch the rest of you. On your feet with your legs slightly more than shoulder-width apart, bend over and place your hands on the floor in front of you. If you're feeling especially limber, move your hands farther back so they're more in line with your heels. You'll feel the stretch in your neck, down your spine, and along your hamstrings. Remember, *don't* bounce this stretch, and keep your stomach pulled in. Hold for a count of thirty.

Move your hands along the floor to your right leg and take hold of your right ankle with your left hand. Reach your right arm straight up, behind you. Hold it there as you count to thirty, working at gently pulling your chest closer to your right leg, all the while holding in your stomach and pulling up on your quads.

After your count of thirty on this leg, gently and slowly move over to repeat the stretch on your left leg. Hold your left ankle with your right hand and keep your left arm raised over your head. Hold on to this stretch for a count of thirty.

Time to go down to the floor and sit for the straddle stretch, with your legs open as wide as they can. Keep your legs down against the floor and your toes pointed upward. Now slowly bend your torso down between your legs, reaching your arms straight out as far as you can in front of you. You'll hold this position for a count of thirty and, as you do, keep trying to increase the stretch by inching your hands forward so your chest is closer to being flat against the floor. (Figure 8.2)

Now slowly move your hands around to your left leg and place your arms on either side of your left leg. Bend gently over your leg, reaching your hands out as far as you can get them. This week, you may be able to grab hold of your foot. As you count to thirty, gently work at getting your chest to lie flat against your leg—or as close to it as possible.

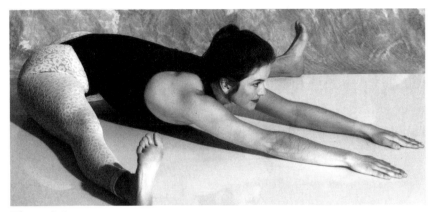

Figure 8.2

When you're through stretching this leg, move your hands across the floor to your right leg and repeat the stretch on this side. Don't bounce, just hold and stretch for a count of thirty.

Now that your muscles feel energized and ready to work, it's time to go to the barre.

First Position

We'll start in First Position with your heels touching, lifted one inch off the floor. Suck in your tummy and tuck your pelvis, knees bent two inches. Roll your shoulders up, back, and down and then keep them squared off like that. Lift your right arm up over your head. Hold on to the barre with your left. You'll stay balanced and your chest will remain open so you're breathing more efficiently.

Start tucking—four times at the first level. Tuck, release but, remember, don't release far—keep those hips forward—tuck, release, tuck, release, tuck, release. Bend your knees another inch and tuck four times here. Bend a third inch and tuck four times.

We're going to plié here like we did last week. So after you tuck four times at the bottom level, plié ten times.

Keep in mind the plié is a small movement. With your knees bent, lower an inch and rise an inch. Lower and rise just one inch each way. Move smoothly, deliberately—down and up ten times. Then go back to the starting position, where your knees are bent two inches, and tuck four times again to start your second repetition.

You'll be doing six repetitions and at the bottom level of each repetition do the ten pliés. After you've completed the first set, check your posture in the mirror. Then move on to a second set of six repetitions with four tucks at each of the three levels and again the ten pliés at the bottom of each repetition.

This week we're adding a third complete set. So right after your last ten pliés, go back up to the first level where you repeat four tucks and lower an inch and do four tucks and lower to the third level and tuck again four times. Now plié ten times and move back up to the first level and repeat the entire set.

By now your quads are screaming to be stretched. This stretch is going to feel good and it will help prepare your thigh muscles for the next strengthening exercise.

We'll start with the Standing Quad Stretch. Bend your knees and tuck your pelvis. Using your right leg as your standing leg, hold the barre with your right hand, bend your left knee and use your left hand to take hold of your left foot up and behind you. Hold on to your foot and gently pull it in toward your seat. Do not touch your seat—instead hold your foot about three inches away from your seat. Now deepen that tuck by squeezing your butt harder and curling forward as far as you can—hips up, butt under. The deeper the tuck, the longer the stretch. Keep an eye on your shoulders. Don't let them round forward. Stand up straight and *fe-e-e-e-e-l* that quad stretch. Hold for a count of twenty.

Now switch standing legs. Turn around and put your left hand on the barre and use your left leg as your standing leg. Again, tuck and bend your right leg back behind you. Holding your right leg with your right hand, gently pull back for the stretch in your right quad. Squeeze that seat and hold for a count of twenty.

Second Position

With your feet shoulder-width apart, lift your heels one inch off the floor. Suck in your tummy and tuck your pelvis. Bend your knees two inches. Check your posture. Lift your chest up so it doesn't rest on your rib cage. Now start your tucking. Do four tucks at the first level, four tucks at the second level, and four at the third level. We're going to add the scoop here.

At the third level down, after you've tucked four times, release slightly, lower slightly, squeeze your butt, scoop under with your pelvis, and reaffirm your tuck. Now lift back up to the third level. Lower, scoop, lift again. Do it four more times and then go back up to the first level and start all over again. You do six repetitions like this: Tuck four times at each level. At the bottom level—each time—lower, scoop, and lift five times. Then return to the first level. Do six of these repetitions to complete one set. Do two sets. (Figure 8.3)

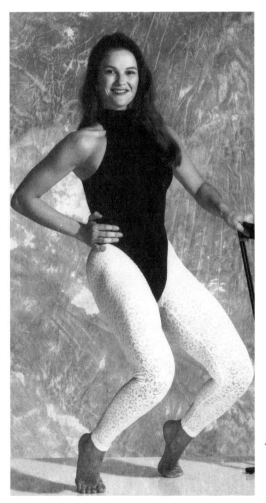

Figure 8.3

Finish up on the floor with the quad stretch. Put your weight on your left knee and move your right leg forward—bending it at the knee. Your toes should point straight ahead. Lean your chest against your right leg and slide your left knee back. Press your left hip forward and down. Reach behind you and lift your left foot with your right hand, pulling it toward your seat. Hold this stretch for a count of ten and switch legs, repeating the stretch on your right leg.

By this week, this stretch should be feeling familiar to your thigh muscles. That's the sign you're really getting them into shape.

Third Position

You'll need the ball for this one. With your feet apart, up on your toes, ball securely between your knees and your knees bent two inches, tuck four times, lower an inch and tuck four times. Lower a third inch and tuck four times. (Figure 8.4)

Now add this movement at the third level: Tuck two times, lower another inch, tuck two times and move back up one inch. Remember, at the third level you're digging deepest into your muscle strength. Do this move three times and then go back up to the first level and start your second repetition. Six repetitions equals one set. Do two sets.

Move on to your full-extension quad stretch. Start with your right leg forward, knee bent. Your left knee is back. Press forward and down with your left hip, then lift your left foot and hold it, stretching your quad for a count of ten. (See Figure 7.6, page 96)

As you lower your left foot to the floor, stretch your left leg back and your right leg forward until it's straight out in front of you. Your elbows are bent slightly on either side of your right leg. Put your nose to your knee and hold for a count of ten. This will really stretch your hamstrings. Be careful *never* to bounce this stretch. Move into it slowly and hold it steadily. Your flexibility is better this week and you're getting your right leg closer to the floor.

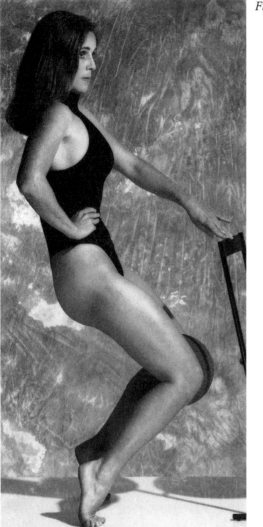

Figure 8.4

After you hold for ten—switch legs—your right foot is back and your left leg is forward. Repeat the quad stretch by holding your right foot behind you for a count of ten. Then move into the hamstring stretch by extending your right foot farther back and straightening your left foot and extending it. Keep your elbows bent slightly and put your nose to your knee and hold for a count of ten.

TWICE UPON A WALL

If you've been sitting a lot or have any tension in your lower back, these next exercises are exceptionally good to relieve the stress and the tightness.

Lie with your feet flat against the wall and your knees bent so that your hips are directly underneath your knees. Place the ball between your knees. Squeeze your seat up and squeeze the ball. Hold for a count of three. Release slightly and squeeze the ball again for a count of three. This week we're adding five more so you'll squeeze up and in a total of twenty times to complete one set. Make sure you don't release your seat. Keep it tilted up and squeezing hard. Start your second set by repeating the tilt and squeeze for a count of three. Do this movement twenty times to complete the second set. (Figure 8.5)

Move right into the next movement, which is to squeeze the ball in, in again, and tilt up. This in, in, up motion counts as one. This week we do it twenty times to complete a set. On the last count, squeeze and hold for a count of ten. Then do two more sets of twenty each—and at the end of each set hold the last squeeze and tilt up for a count of ten.

Now take away the ball but keep your feet and knees shoulder-width apart. This is exactly like last week. Reaffirm your squeezing butt and do the following motion: Up, up, down, down, curling your lower spine up as you go but never lifting your back off the floor. Do twenty cycles of this up, up, down, down motion to complete one set. On the last up motion, squeeze your seat and hold your tuck for a count of ten. Release it and repeat the set.

Now put your knees together and feet together up on the wall. Keep your seat squeezing hard and rotate up one inch and down one inch. This is your count of one. Repeat it twenty times to complete one set. Do two sets of this one inch up and one inch down—always squeezing your knees tightly together. (Figure 8.6)

Stay in the same position and add another movement with your feet together, knees together. Tap your butt gently on the floor two

Figure 8.5

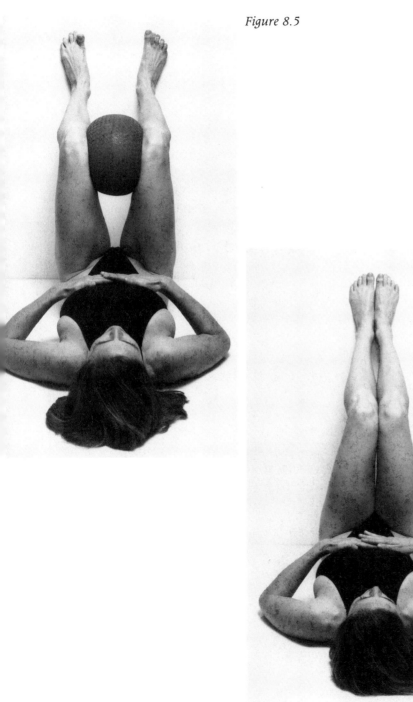

Figure 8.6

times, then curl up—squeezing your seat. Do this tap, tap, curl-up movement twenty times to complete a set. Do two sets.

Hug your knees. You deserve it.

LEG LIFTS

Move away from the wall and lie on your right side. Extend your legs in front of you at a ninety-degree angle to your torso. Make sure your left elbow is planted firmly on the floor parallel to your chest. Tuck your pelvis, release. Tuck, release and tuck and *hold*. Lock in that tuck. It's going to give you strength and it's going to shape your butt. (See Figure 6.10, page 86)

Lift your left leg up and up again—no higher than hip height. If your tuck is set you won't be able to move your leg any higher. Do an up, up, down, down movement fifty times to complete a set. On your last up movement, hold for a count of ten. Then do another set. You'll do three sets of fifty.

Now on your back for the stretch. No matter how strong you are in these leg lifts you'll really feel the stretch—maybe even more than the lifts.

Take your left leg—the one you just worked—and bend it at the knee, cross your left ankle over your right leg, which is up in the air. Now reach through and pull your right leg toward you—stretching the outer thigh of your left leg and your butt. Hold for a count of twenty. Do the same stretch on your right leg. (See Figure 6.9, page 85)

Now lie down on your left side and place your legs at a ninety-degree angle to your torso. This time you'll work the right leg. Up, up, down, down . . . fifty times to a set. Three sets.

Return to your back and stretch your right leg—with your right ankle over your left knee. Pull back on your left leg and hold the stretch for twenty. Repeat it on your left leg.

And then it's time for the cool-down stretch. Stay on your back with both legs bent at the knee, feet flat on the floor. Lift your left leg and reach for it with both hands. Reach for your ankle or foot. Pull your leg as close to your body as possible. Flex your foot and straighten your knee. Lift your head toward the knee. You'll feel the stretch from the back of the knee all the way up to the base of your butt. Hold for a count of thirty. Release and switch. Stretch your right leg. Hold for a count of thirty.

You've done it. Look at yourself in the mirror and tell yourself you're special. Now that you know it, other people will know it, too. And believe us—that feeling tastes richer than any food in the world.

CHAPTER NINE

WEEK SIX

TAKIN' IT TO THE MAX

This is the week we're takin' it to the max. The exercises this week are tough, there's no question about it. But since you've been working diligently, you know all the work up to this point has required fortitude and a strong desire to succeed.

You're very much like many of the models and actresses who come to the studio to work out. They work hard at preparing for their roles, they go out with self-confidence and then when they get what they're after, they work hard at staying on top, constantly improving on what they've achieved. Just like you. You've been rehearsing for your role as the woman with "World Class Legs." This week you're going to take your pursuit as far as it will go. And once you get it down, you're going to keep on improving.

Achieving World Class Legs is a dynamic undertaking. There's never a place where you can be complacent. Happy, yes. Smug, no. World-class contenders never stop striving. And neither should you.

Now that your attitude's heated up, let's warm up your body. Start the music and lift—thirty times with each leg—touching your toes to your hands extended in front of you. Stand tall and proud as you go.

Now move your hands out to the side, shoulder level. Keep those legs lifting. Take your arms up and back to shoulder level. Do another sixty leg lifts while you pump your arms.

Put your hands on your shoulders and plant your feet firmly on the floor. Tuck up that pelvis, good and strong. You know the move here—it's to the side with your torso, back to center, and to the other side. That's a count of one. Do twenty of these and move on to push-ups.

Do two sets of twelve regular push-ups with your knees on the floor and your hands pointing straight out in front of you. Pull in your tummy to protect your back and go down two inches and down two more inches.

Turn your hands in toward each other and do your triceps push-ups. Remember, your weight is on your arms, and your tummy is pulled in. Go down, down, up, up. That's one. Do twelve and then another twelve to complete two sets.

We're going to add a new triceps push-up here. Go over to a sofa or a sturdy chair that won't move. Stand with your back to the front of it. Put your arms behind you and lower yourself, placing your hands on the end of the sofa or chair. Your fingers should be pointed forward so the backs of your arms are parallel to the ceiling and your hands support your body weight on the sofa. Bend your knees in front of you. Now lower your body—but don't drop your butt—down two inches and up two inches. You're working the triceps hard but your biceps get in on this one, too. Do this down, up motion ten times to complete one set. (Figures 9.1 and 9.2)

When you're finished, go for the stretch. Raise your right arm, extending it over your head and then bend it back at the elbow. With your left hand reach up and over your head to your right elbow. Then gently push back and down on your right elbow until you feel the stretch in the back of your arm. Hold for a count of twenty, increasing the stretch as you hold. (See Figure 6.2, page 75)

*   *   *

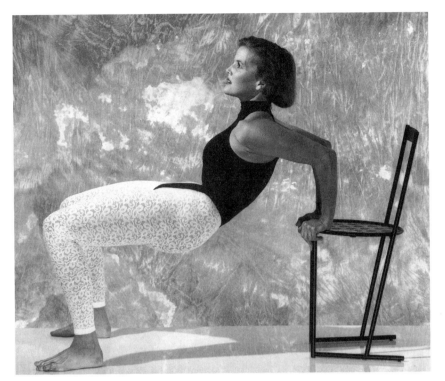

Figure 9.1

Figure 9.2

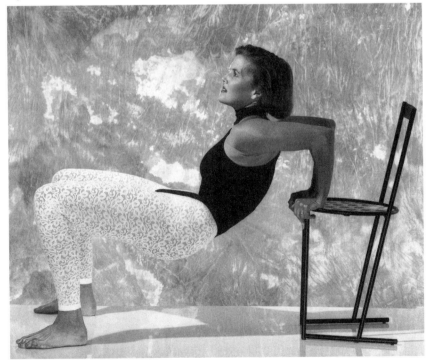

Now stretch your right arm across your body, reaching for the top of your left arm or your shoulder. Use your left hand to grab your right elbow and pull it closer to your chest. You'll feel the stretch in your upper arm. Hold it for a count of twenty.

Repeat both movements with your left arm. First, bend it back behind you and use your right hand to gently push your elbow back and down. Hold for a count of twenty, then stretch your left arm in front of you, extending your left hand as you pull the left elbow closer to your chest with your right hand. Hold this stretch for a count of twenty.

Go back to the first two basic stretches. Start by bending forward and placing your hands on the floor. Pull up on your quads and pull in on your tummy. Keep your hands as close to your feet as possible. Hold for a count of thirty, and then, without moving your hips, move your arms to your left side, pointing your nose to your left knee and grabbing your left ankle with your right hand. Hold your left arm up behind you. Count to thirty and repeat the same stretch on your right leg. (See Figure 7.4, page 93)

Get down on the floor and do your straddle stretches. First, with your legs open wide and your upper body down in between your legs, reach your hands out as far as possible. Hold your torso as close to the floor as you can for a count of thirty and then move over to your left leg for a count of thirty and then over to your right leg for a count of thirty.

With your muscles newly energized and warmed up, you're going to go into First Position at the barre.

UP AT FIRST

While holding on to the barre with one hand, put your heels together and raise them one inch off the floor. Bend your knees two inches and check your posture. Make sure your chest is lifted. Now squeeze your seat into your pelvic tuck. Tuck and release four times at this first level. Drop an inch and tuck and release four more times.

Do the same at the third level—tuck and release four times. Do this descending movement six times to complete one set. Do three sets. (Figure 9.3)

Pick up that ball and place it between your knees. You're still in First Position here. Make sure your knees are bent two inches out over your toes. The pressure of your knees is holding the ball in place. Tuck four times. Now, keeping in the tuck, squeeze the ball four times. Lower another interval and do the same—tuck four times and squeeze four times. Lower to the third level and repeat.

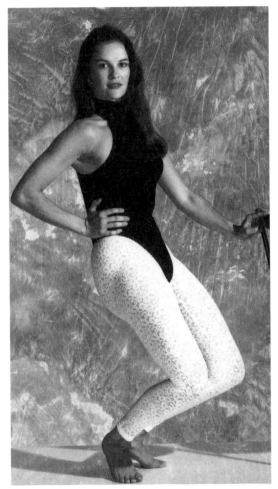

Figure 9.3

Do this tucking and squeezing motion six times to complete a set and then drop the ball and do your standing quad stretch. First, use your right leg as your standing leg and hold your left foot up and behind you for a count of thirty. Then reverse legs and stretch your right quad.

Place the ball back between your knees, holding it securely. Hold on to the barre with your left hand. Hold your right arm up and check your posture—chest up, shoulders back. Beginning with the starting position, slowly lower three counts, scoop your pelvis, and lift. You're squeezing the ball and your seat simultaneously here. The harder you squeeze your butt, the more energy you'll get into your legs. Don't release your seat. Do this lower, scoop, lift motion eight times. Then, at the end, hold in the lower position for a count of ten. Then, rise back up and start your second set of eight repetitions. Again, hold for a count of ten at the bottom of the last repetition.

Now go to the floor and stretch those quads. Put your weight on your left knee and stretch your right leg forward, bending it at the knee. Your toes should point straight ahead. Lean your chest against your right leg and slide your left knee back. Press your left hip forward and down. Reach behind you with your right hand and lift your left foot, pulling it toward your seat. Hold this stretch for a count of ten and switch legs, repeating the stretch on your right leg.

SHIFTING UP TO SECOND

Let's move into Second Position. Your feet are shoulder-width apart. Lift your heels at least one inch off the floor. Suck in your tummy, tuck your pelvis, and bend your knees two inches. Roll your shoulders up, back, and down and lift your chin. (Figure 9.4) Raise your right arm overhead if you can. It will help keep your body lifted—improving your posture.

Start by tucking four times, smoothly move down an inch to the second level and tuck four times. Move one inch down again and tuck four more times.

Figure 9.4

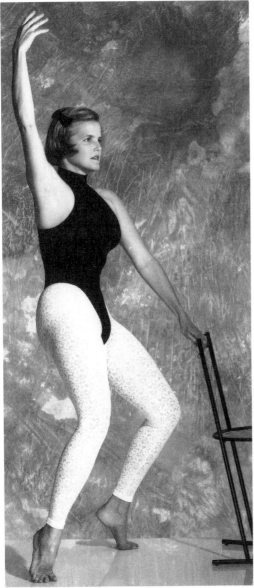

Stay at this bottom level and tuck two more times, then plié—
remember it's that small, smooth movement down one inch. Tuck
two times at this fourth level and smoothly rise up one inch to the
third level. Don't bounce! Your muscles are working hard and deep

here and a bounce won't be as effective. Do this down, tuck, up movement five times, then move back up to the first level and tuck four times to start your second repetition.

Hang in there. . . . Do six repetitions to complete one set. Remember, each time you're at the third level, tuck an extra two times, plié down an inch, tuck twice, and plié up an inch. Do this five times and go back up to the first level.

After this set go back down to the floor and do your quad stretch. First, with your right leg forward, bent at the knee, and your left leg back—with your chest on your right knee, pull your left foot in toward your seat and hold it for a count of ten. Make sure you're squeezing your seat here. Switch legs and stretch your right quad for a count of ten.

MOVING UP TO THIRD

You're getting closer to home plate here, so grab that ball and move into Third Position.

Your feet are apart and parallel, with your knees and toes pointing forward. Place the ball between your knees. All this ball work is strengthening your tendons and ligaments. Grasp the ball with your knees and bend them about two inches. Lift your right heel and then lift your left heel. (Figure 9.5)

Tuck four times at the first level, four times at the second level, and again at the third. Here at the bottom level, after you've tucked four times, squeeze the ball twice and tuck twice. Do this squeeze, squeeze, tuck, tuck two times and go back up to the first level and repeat the entire movement six times to complete one set. Do two of these sets.

Now let's add another set. Tuck four times at the first level and four times at the second and third levels. At the third level, squeeze the ball in and in again, then lower one more inch and squeeze the ball in and in again—then go up one inch and repeat the in, in, lower, in, in, rise movement four times at the end of each repetition. You'll do six repetitions to complete one set here.

*   *   *

Figure 9.5

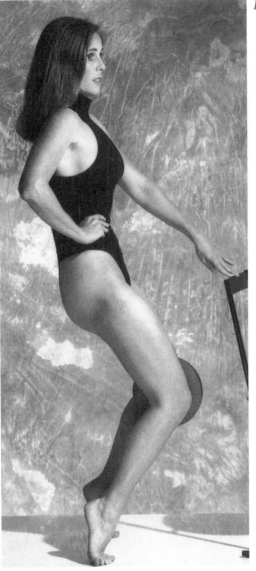

You've been working your quads pretty heavily here. They need to be stretched out, so go to the floor and move on to your full extension quad stretch. Start with your right leg forward, knee bent. Your left knee is back. Press forward and down with your left hip, then lift your left foot and hold it, stretching your quad for a count of ten.

As you lower your left foot back to the floor, stretch your left leg back and your right leg forward until it's straight out in front of you. Your elbows are bent slightly on either side of your right leg. Put your nose to your knee and hold for a count of ten. This will really stretch your hamstrings. Be careful never to bounce this stretch. Move into it slowly and hold it steadily. Your flexibility is better this week and you're getting your right leg closer to the floor.

After you hold for ten, switch legs. Your right foot is back and your left leg is forward. Repeat the quad stretch by holding your right foot behind you for a count of ten. Then move into the hamstring stretch by stretching your right leg farther back and straightening your left leg and extending it. Keep your elbows bent slightly and put your nose to your knee and hold for a count of ten.

You really need to stretch out here so we can keep working on your hamstrings and quads. We're going to do the same straddle stretch that we do in the warm-up.

Sitting on the floor, open your legs as wide as you can. Now lean your torso down between your legs—reaching as far forward as possible with your hands. Keep your legs flat on the floor and your toes pointing up. Hold your stretch here for a count of thirty. Move over to your left leg—gently, slowly—and put your torso down on your left thigh. Keep your arms placed on either side of your leg and reach forward to grasp your foot. This stretch is working your hamstrings and your calf as you pull back on your toes. Stay in this position for a count of thirty, then move over to your other leg and repeat the stretch.

WALL WORK

We're going to increase the wall work this week, and the rewards will really be worthwhile. Not only do these movements shape and strengthen your hamstrings and butt, but they could improve your sex life, too.

The sex muscle (the pubococcygeal, also known as the PC, muscle) stretches from the pubic bone in front, around the genitals on both sides to the tailbone in back. It supports the pelvis and holds internal organs in place.

A weak PC muscle causes a number of medical problems for women—like incontinence and prolapse (falling) of the uterus as well as childbirth problems in general. And women who have weak PC muscles almost never have orgasms. A strong and healthy PC muscle generally means heightened sexual response and pleasure.

Our wall exercises work this muscle along with the inner thighs. And our repetitions act to strengthen the PC muscle along with your legs and butt.

Lie down and put your feet up on the wall, your hips and knees in line and your thighs parallel to the wall. Put the ball between your knees and hold it there securely. Tuck up and release, tuck up and release. Tuck and hold. That's your starting point. Remember to keep your waist on the floor and lift only your butt. (See Figure 8.5, page 117)

Squeeze up and squeeze in on the ball. Hold for a count of three. Release slightly and repeat the motion: Squeeze up and squeeze in on the ball and hold for a count of three. Do this twenty times. On the last count, squeeze and hold the ball for a count of ten. Now return to your original tuck position and reaffirm that tuck.

Squeeze the ball twice and tuck up. So while you're in the tuck position—seat squeezing hard—the rhythm here is in, in, up. Do this twenty times—which is one set—and on the last count squeeze and hold for ten.

Now you're going to repeat the entire combination. Up and squeeze—hold for a count of three. Do it twenty times and on the last count squeeze and hold for ten. Reaffirm your tuck and then repeat the in, in, up motion twenty more times to complete a second set.

After the second set, add an additional set of in, in, up and in, in, down. Do twenty of these movements and finish by squeezing—in the up position—and hold for a count of ten.

You can take away the ball but keep your legs parallel, shoulder-width apart. Now squeeze your seat and tuck up an inch and up another inch, then go down an inch and down another inch. Don't lose your tuck or release your seat. On your last count up hold and squeeze for ten. Then do a second set. (See Figure 6.7, page 83)

Move your feet and your knees together. The movement on this one is: tap your seat gently on the floor two times and then curl up your pelvis. That's a count of one. Do this tap, tap, curl twenty times to complete one set. Do two sets.

Keeping your feet and your knees together, rotate your pelvis up one inch and back down one inch. Don't release your seat. Keep it squeezing. Rotate up one inch, down one inch. Do it twenty times to complete one set. Do two sets.

Hug your knees.

Bring the soles of your feet together, let your knees fall open and pull your feet in as close to your body as possible. This will stretch out your inner thighs. Hold for a count of twenty. Now move away from the wall and get ready for your leg lifts.

THE NONSURGICAL LIFT

Lie on your right side and plant your left elbow firmly in front of you. Bring your legs out in front at a ninety-degree angle to your torso. Tuck and release and tuck and release. Tuck and lock it into place. You're going to work against this tuck as you firm and lift your butt into youthful shape.

Lift your left leg up an inch and up another inch. Bring it down once and down again to the starting position. Do not stop to rest your left leg on your right. Keep it moving up, up, down, down. Do this fifty times with your left leg. Roll to your back and stretch it out.

Cross your left ankle over your right knee and pull back on your right leg to deepen the stretch on the left. Hold for a count of twenty. Repeat the stretch on your other leg. Then switch sides and lie on your left side with your right leg on top. Move your legs into the ninety-degree angle and repeat the up, up, down, down movement fifty times with this leg. Roll onto your back and stretch both legs.

Repeat the entire exercise—fifty lifts with each leg—and repeat the stretch.

*   *   *

Go back into the ninety-degree-angle position, starting on your right side with your left leg on top. Rotate your pelvis. Lift your left leg to starting position at hip height. Lock your knee into place, squeeze your seat, and lift your left leg one inch. Lower it one inch. Do this smoothly ten times. Pause. Move your leg forward one inch and back one inch. Do this ten times. Now combine one inch up, back down to center, one inch forward and back to center. One up, one forward equals one repetition. Do ten of these to complete one set. Repeat the whole cycle. (Figure 9.6)

Stretch your left leg by crossing your left ankle over your right knee. Hold the stretch for a count of twenty. Go directly to your left side with your right leg on top. Repeat the exercise with your right leg.

Now stretch your right leg by crossing your right ankle over your left knee. Pull back on your left leg to deepen the stretch. Hold for a count of twenty.

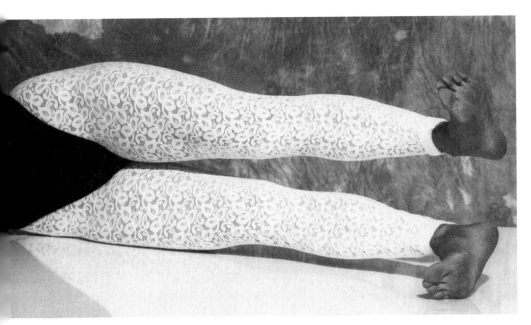

Figure 9.6

COOLING DOWN—BUT NOT OFF

That was quite some job you did. Now let's do our one last stretch for the day.

Stay on your back with both legs bent at the knee, feet flat on the floor. Lift your left leg and reach for it with both hands.

Reach for your ankle or foot. Pull your leg as close to your body as possible. Flex your foot and straighten your knee. Lift your head toward the knee. You'll feel the stretch from the back of the knee all the way up to the base of your butt. Hold for a count of thirty. Release and switch. Stretch your right leg. Hold for a count of thirty.

You've just completed a World Class Workout. And you've done a terrific job. The exercises you've been mastering these past six weeks will change the shape of your legs, thighs, and butt. But you have to remain diligent. Keep up the routine. Do it at least three times a week. You can either repeat Week Six as it appears in this chapter or you can get creative and combine different moves from any of the other weeks' routines. You can always increase the repetitions or the levels at which you work.

Reaffirm your tuck and you're reaffirming your self-worth. Remember, your exercise time is a precious investment. You have to make regular deposits to cash in on the dividends.

Your body is the account. You're investing your workout time, and your improved self-esteem pays off with a big bonus. With World Class Legs, the interest's in you. Keep up the good work!

CHAPTER TEN

TAKIN' IT ON THE ROAD

Exercise is as vital to your well-being as breathing, eating, and sleeping. So if you're setting off to breathe, eat, and sleep somewhere other than home, pack up your exercises and take them with you. You don't need much room in either your suitcase or your day.

In addition to this book, take a leotard or a pair of tights and a T-shirt. Pack one of your exercise music tapes and your Walkman (they also make portable speakers that can easily be tucked into your bag) and bring a tennis ball that's a little mushy.

You're probably on a tight schedule—especially if you're on a business trip—but you'll find if you take the fifteen or twenty minutes to do this "quickie" workout you'll feel more energized the rest of the day. And you can do it right in your hotel room or guest room.

LET THE MUSIC PLAY

Turn on the music. Your body will respond to the rhythm automatically. Take a few deep breaths and start your warm-up. Lift those legs to your arms, extended from your shoulders. Lift thirty times with each leg. Keep lifting and move your arms out to the side—shoulder level—then up overhead and back to center. Lift another sixty times here—thirty with each leg.

Now, with both feet firmly on the floor, bend your knees two inches and put your hands on your shoulders. Bend from the waist—to the side, back up to center, and down to the other side. That's one. Do this twenty times.

Down to the floor for push-ups. You're on your knees, weight shifted forward on your arms, fingers pointed straight ahead. Go down, down, then up, up. Do these regular push-ups ten times and then turn your hands in toward each other and do ten triceps push-ups . . . down, down, up, up.

Move right into your body stretch. Feet shoulder-width apart, bend your knees, lean forward with your hands on the floor, straighten your knees and hold for a count of thirty. Without moving your hips, bring your nose to your left knee, right hand to left ankle, left arm up over your head and stretch. Hold for thirty. Move to your right leg and repeat the stretch.

Get down on the floor and do your straddle stretch. First, bend your torso down between your legs and reach forward with your arms. Hold for a count of thirty. You'll get more flexible throughout the stretch.

Slowly move to your left leg. Place your chest on your thigh and your arms on either side of your leg. Reach to your ankle or your foot if you can and hold this stretch for a count of thirty. Then slowly move over to your right leg and repeat the stretch.

BELLY UP TO THE BARRE

Use a chair or table as your barre. Remember, the barre should be about hip high. Hold on to it lightly and move into First Position, heels together and lifted one inch off the floor, suck in your tummy, tuck in your pelvis, bend your knees two inches to starting position.

Tuck four times, lower an inch and tuck four times, and lower an inch to the third level and tuck four times and then *hold* for a count of ten.

If you're strong enough, plié four times at the bottom level. The plié is that small, smooth movement—down an inch and up an inch. Then you return to the first level.

Do a set of ten. If you've got the time and have built up the strength, do a second set in First Position.

Do a standing quad stretch here. Your right leg is your standing leg. Bend it slightly and tuck your pelvis by squeezing your seat. Take your left foot behind you in your left hand and with your knee bent, pull up and back on your left foot. You're pulling against the tuck. Check your posture. Make sure your chest is lifted high. Hold for a count of twenty. Switch legs and repeat the stretch with your right leg.

Move right into Second Position. Your feet are shoulder-width apart and your heels are one inch off the floor. Suck in your tummy, tuck your pelvis, and bend your knees two inches out over your toes.

Tuck and release four times at the first level, drop an inch and tuck and release four times. Remember: Do not release your tuck completely, just a slight movement and then back into a tighter tuck. Tuck and release four times at the third level down. Then *hold* for a count of ten. That's one. Go back up to the first level and repeat this movement ten times to complete a set.

If you have the time and feel strong enough, do a second set of ten and at the bottom of each repetition substitute four pliés for the hold.

Now let's move into Third Position. Your feet are apart and parallel. Your toes point forward. Tuck your pelvis. Bend your knees out over your toes two inches, and lift your left heel up and then lift your right heel up. Tuck four times at each level here and hold for a count of ten at the bottom level. Do ten repetitions.

You've worked your quads hard since your last stretch, so this time let's do the quad stretch on the floor. Go down on your left knee with your right leg forward, bent at the knee, toes pointed ahead. Put your chest down on your right knee and slide your left knee back. Press your left hip forward and down. Lift your left foot and reach around with your right hand to hold it for a count of ten. Release and switch legs.

UP AGAINST THE WALL

Lie on your back with your feet up on the wall, your hips and knees in line. Put the tennis ball between your knees and hold it there securely. Now rotate your pelvis up—keeping your waist on the floor. Squeeze the ball and hold and squeeze for a count of three. Release the tension slightly and squeeze again for a count of three. Do this twenty times to complete a set. Do two sets and then hug your knees. (Figure 10.1)

THE RIGHT ANGLE ON LEGS

Move away from the wall and lie on your right side. Bring your legs out at a right angle to your torso. Plant your left arm firmly in front of you. Tuck that pelvis and lock it in. Don't release it throughout this entire exercise. If you feel the tuck slipping, stop and reaffirm.

Now lift your left leg up, up, then take it down, down. It should not go above hip level and on the bottom it should not rest. Keep it moving—fluidly—for fifty counts. On the last lift *hold* for a count of ten. Then repeat a second set of fifty.

Take a minute here to stretch out your outer thigh and butt. Roll over onto your back and cross your left ankle over your right knee. Your right leg is extended in the air and you reach and pull it back toward you—stretching your left outer thigh for a count of twenty.

Now lie on your left side, bring your legs out at a right angle, plant your front arm firmly, tuck your pelvis and do fifty leg lifts up, up,

Figure 10.1

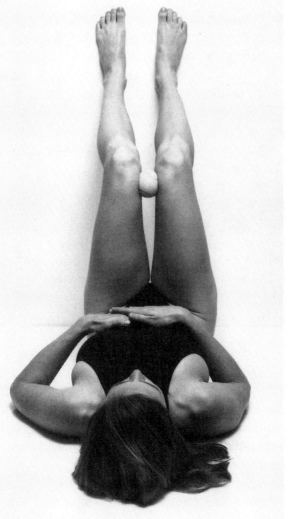

down, down. Hold for a count of ten on the last lift. Repeat the set.

Stretch out your right outer thigh and your butt by crossing your right ankle over your left knee and pulling back on your left leg. Hold for a count of twenty.

Let's cool down with our cool-down stretch. You're on your back. Bend both legs at the knee, feet flat on the floor. Lift your left leg and reach for it with both hands. Reach as high as you can—anywhere from below your knee to your ankle or even your foot. Pull your leg as close to your body as possible. Make sure your tummy is pulled in. Flex your foot and straighten your knee. Lift your head toward the knee. You'll feel the stretch all along the back of your leg up to your butt. Hold for a count of thirty. Switch legs and repeat.

You should be feeling pretty energized by now, and with this workout completed, you've already accomplished something for the day. You're stretched for success!

ANYTIME, ANYWHERE

You can do certain of our exercises anytime, anywhere. Here are a few examples. If you're standing in line at the supermarket or at the bank, gently tuck your pelvis and squeeze and release your butt as many times as you can.

You can squeeze and release to your heart's content when you're standing in the kitchen cutting vegetables or when you're watching TV or driving somewhere in the car.

If you work at a desk, keep a mushy tennis ball in your bottom drawer and at least once a day, sit at the edge of your chair with the tennis ball between your knees and squeeze and release thirty times.

Whenever you get up out of a chair, start by lifting your shoulders up, rolling them back and down.

Always remember to keep your tummy pulled in. It will help your posture; it will protect your back and you'll look longer and leaner, too. Eventually a tighter, flatter tummy will be yours naturally.

When you go to the ladies' room, take a couple of extra minutes to stretch. Bend your knees and then bend your torso forward, reaching for the floor (take off your high heels, of course). Reach over to your left leg and stretch, then your right leg. You'll get the blood flowing, you'll loosen your spine, and you'll stretch those hamstrings. All part of a day's work. In fact, it will improve your day's work.

Be creative about finding a time and place to tuck and stretch. Remember, don't do anything strenuous without a warm-up. The more time you spend doing your workout, the more in touch with your body you'll become. And the more you get used to our movements the easier it will be for you to be flexible with them.

No matter where your World Class Legs take you, stand proud and tall and top them off with a World Class Smile.

AUTHOR BIOS

Felix Schmitt is turning Hollywood into the capital of World Class Legs. As trainer to the stars, including Michelle Pfeiffer and Dyan Cannon and cover girls Christy Turlington and Kim Henderson, among others, Felix has taught thousands of women how to have World Class Legs at his exclusive West Hollywood studio: Sunset Plaza Fitness. He's developed an exercise method for women of the '90s that has successfully shaped the legs and butts of women of all ages.

Cynthia Tivers is a Hollywood-based writer and television-producer, and director. Among the many series she's worked on are "Good Morning America"; "Lifestyles of the Rich and Famous"; and "PM Magazine." She's also written, directed, and produced a number of television specials, including the "Mrs. America" and "Mrs. World" pageants, "The Best of L.A.," and "Inner City Games . . . Ticket to Life." Ms. Tivers is a graduate of Northwestern University's Medill School of Journalism and she's been a student at Sunset Plaza Fitness for five years.